Dynamic Positions
in Birth

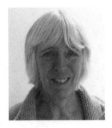

About the author

Ever since the birth of her third child in 1991, Margaret Jowitt has been working towards making birth a safer and more rewarding experience for mothers and their babies. After a first degree in music and psychology, she gained an MPhil from Keele in 1998, researching into Mothers' Experience of Birth at Home and in Hospital.

Her first book, *Childbirth Unmasked*, published in 1993, looked at the anatomy and physiology of birth, showing how stress hormones conflict with birth hormones. Since 1996 she has edited *Midwifery Matters*, the magazine of the Association of Radical Midwives. She considers that prevention is better than cure and believes that good midwifery care based on the needs of the individual woman is the key to safer childbirth.

Dynamic Positions in Birth

A fresh look at how women's bodies work in labour

Margaret Jowitt

2nd edition

Dynamic Positions in Birth: A fresh look at how women's bodies work in labour

First published in Great Britain by Pinter & Martin Ltd 2014
This 2nd edition published 2020

ISBN 978-1-78066-690-7

British Library Cataloguing-in-Publication Data
A catalogue record for this book is available from the British Library.

Editor Debbie Kennett

Index Helen Bilton

Author photograph John Nash

Set in Minion

Printed and bound by Hussar, Poland

This book has been printed on paper that is sourced and harvested from sustainable forests and is FSC accredited.

Pinter & Martin Ltd
6 Effra Parade
London SW2 1PS

www.pinterandmartin.com

Contents

In memory of HMO and JHS

Preface

There has been rather a long gap between this book and my last. *Childbirth Unmasked* (1993) dealt with the adverse effect of stress on labour. Relaxation had been known to help women cope with labour since Grantly Dick-Read's book *Childbirth without Fear* in the 1940s. I wanted to know the physiological mechanisms underlying the perception that labour was less painful and progressed better at home and found that stress hormones down-regulated labour hormones. I came to the conclusion that stress hormones regulate labour hormones according to the mother's stress, slowing things down when the mother is stressed. Also in that book I started to think about how the uterus worked. I mentioned the mother's position only in passing but the seeds were laid for this present book which complements the first. Getting into the right position played a large part in the labours and births of three of my four babies.

Childbirth Unmasked came out just before the *Changing Childbirth* report in 1993 which was supposed to improve birth for all women. Everyone in the childbirth movement had high hopes that at long last childbirth would change. But instead, in the intervening years, the caesarean section rate soared, more and more women opted for an epidural and some avoided labour altogether by choosing surgical delivery. And yet there has been little improvement in the perinatal mortality rate (the number of babies stillborn or dying in the first week of life). I've spent the last 18 years editing *Midwifery Matters*, the magazine of the Association of Radical Midwives, and this has added to my wider knowledge of birth. The stories of women giving birth under midwifery care are so very different from the agonising scenes portrayed on our TV screens. When *One Born Every Minute* was screened, I found myself begging the midwives to get women off the bed. I started thinking about designing a piece of furniture to encourage women to labour in different positions and began this book while developing the chair. The book was finished first and now the kneeling chair is tested and available.

As I found with my last book, the more deeply I looked into the clinical research and the physiology, the less sense there seemed to be in the way women usually give birth in our culture. This time round I had the benefit of the internet which gave me access to far more material. I found an ever-widening gulf between physiological science and medical practice. Midwifery practice tends to work with women's physiology. Medical practice has been led astray by well intentioned but ultimately harmful technology which puts a physical and psychological barrier between the labouring woman and those who care for her. I hope this book will help to break down barriers and give women the freedom to move during labour that I was lucky enough to have. I believe that they and their babies will be the better for it.

Preface to the second edition

In 2016 I discovered a biophysical mechanism that could transform a quiescent uterus into one ready for labour. The deafening silence that greeted me after the hypothesis was aired in the *British Journal of Obstetrics and Gynaecology* (Jowitt, 2018) only goes to show what an enormous chasm there is between standard medical practice and what women actually need to labour well. A little while later I learnt that most of the clitoris is hidden inside the body and realised that internal clitoral stimulation was likely to be the trigger for the fetal ejection reflex. These two discoveries meant that a second edition was needed. Mothers and babies both play an active part in birth. Both need to be able to move.

1 Introduction

Birth is an earthquake of an event in a woman's life. Her body experiences the greatest upheaval it has undergone since she herself was born and her psyche gains another layer of womanhood. She is transformed into a mother – a 24/7 job for the next few years. Every baby is a miracle. Every birth is miraculous. We can't get away from the fact that birth is undoubtedly an 'animal' event, but an event so significant that it acquired cultural meaning from the very beginnings of human consciousness. For hundreds of thousands of years birth was a woman's business, taking place in the domestic setting. The labouring woman was surrounded by family members and women with experience of birth and a gift for supporting women in labour, for consciousness brought with it the fear of death and the need for emotional support. Consciousness led to the need for the rituals of religion, a way of dealing with the fears conjured up by the unpredictability of the forces of nature, birth being a prime example.

For millennia the physical, emotional and spiritual needs of a woman giving birth were intertwined but after the mind/body split enunciated in the philosophy of Descartes in the first half of the seventeenth century there was an increasing tendency to see the body as a machine, with faults which could be remedied or bypassed mechanically. Sometimes they could. The invention of the obstetrical forceps brought first man-midwives and then doctors into the birth room. Men of science started to challenge the authority of the Church. The doctor was to become the expert, the midwife to become his assistant. It took 250 years for doctors to gain supremacy over midwifery education with the passing of the *Midwives Act* in 1902 and another 70 years before hospital birth was recommended for all (Short Report, 1970) but the midwifery profession continues to advocate a role for emotional support (Association of Radical Midwives, 2013) and even spirituality (Hall, 2000) and organisations such as the Association for Improvements in the Maternity Services and the National Childbirth Trust carry on campaigning for holistic care in childbirth).

Twentieth-century mainstream obstetrics is predicated entirely upon Cartesian principles and pays only lip service to the emotional aspects of birth. The few obstetricians who attempt to practise a more woman-centred approach risk professional isolation (Savage, 2007; Morrow, 2013). The mind/body split in medicine led directly to the current obstetric view that describes childbirth by means of the powers (the muscular force of the uterus), the passage (the bony pelvis) and the passenger (the fetus). While obstetrics acknowledges that women should have the continuous presence of a midwife, the role of the midwife is chiefly to observe, monitor and call for obstetric help should labour deviate from numerical norms such as the rate of dilatation of the cervix, fetal heart rate patterns, maternal pulse rate or temperature. Machines can now record many of these things; midwives are required to record the rest on the partogram, a chart of progress in labour. In the modern large-scale birth factory system, the midwife becomes a machine minder in the eyes of the management team and is employed on a shift system – any midwife will do. Midwives facing Fitness to Practise hearings at their regulatory body, the Nursing and Midwifery Council (NMC), find themselves faced with lists of shortcomings based on their failure to follow guidelines based on obstetric numerology. Sometimes a successful defence can be mounted in terms of the 'informed refusal' of the woman but even then midwives can face accusations that they did not try hard enough to convince women of the folly of their choices. Apart from the requirement to give respectful and dignified care, the emotional aspects of support in labour are underrated; until *Better Births* in 2016, commissioners of maternity care in the UK resisted calls for continuity of care from a known midwife, despite evidence showing that clinical outcomes are improved (Weston, 2014).

The natural childbirth movement tends to focus its attention on midwifery care in birth centres and at home because these are the places where women – mothers and midwives – are still largely in control of birth, but only 2.5% of women give birth at home and another 5% choose freestanding birth centres. Women who have experienced this type of care cannot speak highly enough of its benefits to themselves and their babies; it eases the transition to motherhood and leads to far less surgical intervention (Birthplace Study Collaboration Team, 2011). At least half of all women are at low risk of complications and could give birth in such places but such is the fear that has been generated around birth that most choose obstetric units.

Despite the clinical and economic benefits of midwifery care shown by the Birthplace Study, the organisation of maternity care in the UK is unlikely to change any time soon and it is time to consider the needs of women choosing to labour in hospital, where the vast majority of women give birth. The western birth culture takes women out of a comfortable place where they make their own rules (home) and turns them into patients in hospital, a place dominated by rules and regulations, policies, protocols and guidelines produced by people wanting to control the behaviour of staff and 'patient' alike. In hospitals care is organised according to medical protocols required by the Clinical Negligence Scheme for Trusts (CNST) which is the 'insurance' arm of the NHS. Maternity hospitals are getting larger and larger as smaller units merge and in these straitened economic times there is pressure to make the most efficient use of bed space in the delivery suite and postnatal ward.

The hospital environment depicted in TV programmes such as *One Born Every Minute* seems very stark to any woman who has laboured and given birth at home or in a birth centre under the care of a midwife. One aspect seems particularly problematic – the bed takes centre stage. Women were not designed by evolution to labour and give birth propped up semi-sitting or lying on their backs. The hospital bed can turn a healthy active woman who is quite capable of trusting her body to give birth by itself into a passive patient hooked up to machines which immobilise her and increase her pain. The obstetric bed dominates the labour room in delivery suites up and down the country and although midwives are well aware of the need to get women off the bed, it is easier said than done when the only alternatives are a large plastic gym ball, a bean bag and perhaps a floor mat. The problem is also one of expectations: women expect to use the bed, and some midwives prefer them to be on it. In fact, labour and birth in any position other than on the bed is usually described as 'alternative'. There is no reason why the bed should not be used mainly for its original purpose – for sleeping – and when necessary for clinical examination. It is easier for a midwife to palpate the abdomen to ascertain the position of the fetus when a woman is supine but labour is easier for women when they can move around freely. Despite its claim to be based on science, the hospital approach to birth knows virtually nothing about the two major influences on how women's bodies work in childbirth – her state of mind and how she and her baby move in the bony spaces that nature has provided.

I find myself in the somewhat paradoxical position of being intensely fascinated by the minutiae of the anatomy and physiology of birth while at the same time believing that birth is best viewed holistically. I believe that the birth of a baby through the extraordinarily shaped human pelvis is an instinctive process written deep into our genes and that the hospital culture both denies and disrupts the instinctive process. This is the behaviour that is elicited during birth when there is no outside interference to disrupt the process as it unfolds – when there is no expectation of labouring on a bed, when there are no machines impeding instinctive movement.

In my last book I considered the hormones of birth and the effect of the psychological environment; in this one I concentrate on the biomechanics of birth. Having accused obstetrics of having too mechanistic a view of birth, I hope I can escape accusations of being a Cartesian dualist myself by including maternal instinct in biomechanics; one cannot argue from science without adopting some of its principles and nothing but an argument from science has any hope of changing anything in that temple of scientific medicine, the hospital. I think we need to go back to first principles, to strip away the cultural paraphernalia that surrounds birth and return to basic biology, anatomy and physiology.

Problems in human childbirth are attributed to upright walking and having to give birth to a baby with too large a head. Evolutionary theorists call this the obstetric dilemma; 'Nature is a bad obstetrician', they say. Are they right? We all know that birth is not always a success story. I once saw a photograph of the skeletal remains of a failed breech birth. The mother and child were buried together with the fetal head still inside the maternal pelvis. The large head only just fits through the pelvis and birth is usually safer when the head is leading the way. Natural breech birth is usually possible but becomes more difficult when attempted under laboratory conditions in hospital; the obstetric solution is to bypass the pelvis and deliver by caesarean section.

We can all be grateful that modern surgery has the means to rescue nature's mistakes but has the female body become so dysfunctional that it can no longer give birth even to babies coming head first through a healthy normal pelvis? Natural selection – the survival and reproduction of the fittest – must have solved each problem as it arrived or we wouldn't be here. Until very recently all humans had to pass through the bottleneck of the female pelvis to be born and, for breastfeeding mammals, survival after birth is heavily dependent upon the survival of the mother, so the vast majority of our great-great-great… grandmothers lived to tell the tale. We have the 'right' genes for successful birth. Whatever convolutions and contortions the body went through on its way to its current form, women evolved to give birth and survive the experience. So why has it all gone so wrong? Today 25% of women in the UK, the country with the best nationalised health service in the world, have to give birth by caesarean section and another 12% with the help of forceps or vacuum extraction.

According to current medical opinion, today's rising caesarean section rate is the consequence of mothers leaving it later to have their first child and maternal obesity. Did evolution 'weed out' older and larger mothers in the past? But older and larger mothers can't account for all today's extra caesareans, and the perinatal mortality rate (the proportion of babies stillborn or not surviving the first week of life) has not fallen commensurately with the rising caesarean rate.

I have been lucky enough to have given birth to four children without any problem and in three of those births it was readily apparent that I needed to adopt a particular position either during the labour or for the birth itself: sitting, squatting, kneeling – and even lying on my side on a bed. Most of these positions weren't to be found in obstetric textbooks although there was much talk about them in the midwifery and childbirth literature. Three positions were labelled 'alternative'. I decided to investigate further and found that there is so much more movement involved in birth than I could have thought possible, and yet so little of it is to be found in the textbooks. Starting from an intuitive instinct derived from my own experience and reinforced by watching such TV programmes as *One Born Every Minute*, I reached a deeper understanding of how the body works in labour.

The illustrations in textbooks are largely limited to an obstetrician's eye view of the mother – or rather parts of her, her uterus and her pelvis. At first they made the problem appear insurmountable – I started to get a real feel for the obstetric dilemma. Unlike other mammals, our babies do not have a direct tunnel from their mother's abdomen to the outside world – our babies have to negotiate a 120-degree bend. This was the core of the obstetric problem but textbooks gave no clues as to how humankind had solved it in deep history. It was time to investigate the anthropological literature and look at what happens in other cultures. Sheila Kitzinger, the doyenne of childbirth anthropology, quoted Jamaican midwives saying that women have to 'open their backs' to give birth (Kitzinger, 1993). Opening the back implies making more space in the pelvis, making more room for a baby to move through it. But opening the back also destabilises the pelvis – the legs can no longer be trusted to support the weight of the body. For the moment of birth itself perhaps we need to become quadrupeds again for a little while; we need the weight of our body to be supported by something other than just our legs. Humans thus appear to need physical support as well as emotional support in birth – our bodies need to be supported in positions which will make that journey easier for us and our babies.

This rang bells for me. Twenty years ago, when my second son was a few days old, I moved awkwardly and put my back out. My legs and pelvis would no longer support my body weight; I needed to use my arms as well. Pregnancy and birth had loosened my pelvic joints and they had not yet returned to pre-pregnancy stability; a sudden awkward movement destabilised my pelvis. Luckily a previous job working for *Physiotherapy* journal had given me the knowledge to seek out a physiotherapist as soon as possible. She realigned the joint and I had no further problems for twenty years. To understand human childbirth we need to explore the function of the pelvis, beginning with the changes to the pelvis that occurred in the journey from walking on all fours to walking on two legs and exploring the means by which the baby might negotiate the bend in the pelvis.

How can a woman's back 'open' if she is lying on it? Women didn't always give birth on their backs. In Europe and in the USA they used to give birth on a birthing stool. The gradual transformation of the birthing stool, a midwifery tool, into the obstetric bed directly mirrors the gradual transcendence of obstetrics over midwifery. A simple portable device carried to the mother's home by a midwife gradually evolved into an obstetric bed designed for operative delivery. The birth itself is the most dramatic part of labour and specialist furniture, high- or low-tech, was designed to help someone do their job, whether it was the mother, the midwife or the obstetrician. The transformation of the birthing stool into the obstetric bed involved a move from home to hospital. The modern obstetric bed has been specifically designed for childbirth in hospital and yet (if the Jamaican midwives are right) it takes no account of a woman's need to open her back. Birth chairs were standard equipment from ancient Egypt right up until the middle of the nineteenth century but as more and more doctors became involved in birth they were forgotten. As far as the physiology of birth was concerned, this was a bit like forgetting the invention of the wheel – or was it? Even a chair restricts the movement of the pelvis.

Providing beds for labour is a historical accident. It is the consequence of sending women to hospital for birth. Hospitals revolve around providing beds for patients, and they measure their capacity in 'beds'. If you hospitalise a woman for the second stage of labour, the birth itself, you have to hospitalise her for the first stage as well. You have to advise her to come in when she is having regular painful contractions, so many minutes apart and lasting so long (the numerology at work again). Even if you advise her to stay at home for as long as possible, she would rather get to a safe place in time for the birth than risk giving birth away from the medical attention that she is told she and her baby need for safety. Anyway travelling in advanced labour is distinctly uncomfortable, so women will arrive sooner rather than later and if labour is advanced enough they will be given a room with a bed in it and a midwife to look after them. And if there is a bed in the room they expect to use it, particularly if they have learned what to expect during labour by watching main channel TV programmes. (They will also expect labour to be excruciatingly painful.) Perhaps scriptwriters have based their scenarios on this:

'Conventional' childbirth. In this choice, the woman is admitted to the maternity ward … She is content to leave the process of childbirth in the care of the obstetric team, and to accept, without question, their management. … She is cared for with skill but *does not participate* in the process of childbirth. (Llewellyn-Jones, 1990) (my italics)

The caesarean section rate has doubled in the UK since this was written, although three years later *Changing Childbirth* (DoH, 1993) was to recommend that women should participate in childbirth: 'the woman should be made the centre of her care' and there have been numerous initiatives to normalise birth but none has worked. The latest reorganisation of the NHS was brought in under the mantra of: 'No decision about me without me' but doesn't always appear to apply to childbirth in hospital. The Birthrights survey of 2013 found that 11% of respondents overall considered that they had not been given information about each examination or procedure before it had been performed; this figure rose to 24% for women having forceps or vacuum (ventouse) deliveries.

Doctors and midwives were trained to 'deliver' women on beds but why should it be assumed that a bed is needed for the first stage of labour, when the cervix is opening up? Lying on a bed for labour is a relatively recent practice largely restricted to hospitals. For millennia midwives helped women cope with labour and give birth in their own homes, from cave to cottage, from tenement to suburban semi. If a mother called a midwife too early it was no big deal for the midwife to go away and do her antenatal clinic or do her postnatal visits and come back later. And even if a woman did end up in her bedroom to give birth on a bed, because that was how midwives were trained to 'deliver', she went there only when the birth was imminent. Once a woman has been admitted to hospital there is nothing for her to do but to be a 'patient' and await the birth of her child. There is nothing to distract her from the pain. (As I write this my gaze alights on the second edition of a book entitled *Active Management of Labour* (O'Driscoll and Meagher, 1986), and it seems ironic that the cover picture is of a woman lying on her left side in bed being touched by a nurse, nothing very active about that. A quick internet search search showed me the cover picture of the fourth edition (2003), a woman in bed, head and shoulders raised on pillows, touching the arm of a nurse. The obstetric bed has become standard equipment for every maternity hospital room in the UK but it turns the labouring mother into a passive patient. It is difficult to see someone confined to bed as doing any work at all. The 'message' of the obstetric bed is that a labouring woman is sick and needs people to do things to her to enable her baby to be born.

Unless you consider a woman's needs for labour separately from her needs for giving birth (or rather the doctor's needs for delivering a baby), you are almost guaranteed to increase her pain by restricting her physical movement and placing limits on her creature comforts – at home she has her own space, her sofa, her kitchen worktops, her bath, her shower. You are also restricting her physical activity. She can't make a cup of tea, and you are denying her the chance to act on her nest-building instincts and scrub the kitchen floor or clean the oven. She can't do the washing up in hospital, and she can't take her ironing board in with her. She can't carry on with life as normal, stopping in her tracks and finding a handy place to lean on as a contraction makes itself manifest. Not only do such activities offer a welcome distraction from labour but they play a part in finding comfortable positions for the mother and, more to the point, they have a chance of optimising the baby's position for the journey to the outside world.

However much hospitals try to create a welcoming atmosphere, clinical concerns about infection control and safety must take priority in the high-risk environment of a hospital. Delivery rooms have become stark, unfriendly places with no soft furnishings – apparently even pillows are nearly always in short supply. As well as the state-of-the-art obstetric bed, the room is full of machines, wires, tubes and buzzers and, of course, the clock looms large. Faced with all these reminders of what can go wrong, and with nothing to do except to wait for the next contraction, it is not surprising that pain becomes an overriding sensation.

The body is working hard during labour and contractions can be very painful – sometimes agonising pain that is very difficult to cope with and requires pain relief, or even anaesthesia which removes all sensation. In the 1930s Grantly Dick-Read hypothesised that there was a fear/tension/pain cycle, saying that pain becomes worse because we expect and fear it and so we become tense, actually causing the pain, a vicious circle. Relaxation for childbirth was introduced and it helped many women, but relaxation alone is not enough to extinguish the pain. It will not remove the sensations of labour. The uterus is doing the amazing job of pushing the baby down to be born and hard work is often accompanied by pain. Restricting women to the bed compels them to adopt positions that prevent their bodies from working as evolution intended, making labour more painful than necessary. During pregnancy, as the baby grows, the main body of the uterus stretches up out of the pelvis, leaving only the cervix in the pelvis. During labour the baby moves down into the pelvis, opening the cervix and stretching everything as he goes, which is bound to be uncomfortable, particularly if the mother is confined to bed and unable to move her pelvis to accommodate him.

In my first book I looked at the interactions between stress hormones and labour hormones. This entailed finding out how the uterus worked, what made it work more efficiently, and what might stop it working. I uncovered intricate relationships between stress hormones and labour hormones and this accounted for some of the differences between labouring under midwifery care and labouring in the high-stress environment of a hospital. I also learnt about the stretch-contract reflex which appears to have some influence on how and where contractions happen in the uterus. I surmised that the uterus needs to be free from external constraints, particularly the mother's spine, in order to contract efficiently and effectively to steer the baby towards the exit. Twenty years on there is much more evidence on how the uterus works and medical physics departments are building up a much fuller picture of contraction patterns using more sophisticated medical imaging. This evidence casts doubt on current teaching about the source and direction of the contractions of the uterus in labour.

Women need physical support in labour as well as emotional support. Adopting different positions for labour will not preclude all the procedures women have come to expect in hospital, such as epidural anaesthesia or electronic fetal monitoring, but it may well prevent much of the intervention that has become commonplace and so often leads to birth by forceps, ventouse and emergency caesarean section. Women should be able to choose to remain active in labour even when doctors want more monitoring. Women need to adopt whatever position they find most comfortable, be it standing, kneeling, leaning, sitting or even lying. Women need furniture to support them in physiologically productive positions for both labour and birth. This is not just for their own comfort but so that they can labour and give birth to their babies in the way that nature intended and give their babies the best possible start in life.

2 Birth furniture through the ages

How did women give birth before we invented furniture? How do other primates cope with labour and birth? Most monkey births occur at night but Ding, Yang and Xiao (2013) observed a daytime birth of a snub-nosed monkey. The mother climbed up a rhododendron tree, faintly calling. After ten minutes her calls turned into screams, and an experienced female black snub-nosed monkey climbed up to the screaming mother. As the baby monkey began to crown, the experienced female sat beside the mother. The actual birth took four and a half minutes. The head, once fully exposed, was grabbed by the midwife monkey who pulled the baby out with both hands. The baby monkey was born in the caul, still enclosed in the membranes. The midwife monkey ripped open the birth membranes, the new mother reclaimed the infant within a minute, and severed the umbilical cord. She ate the placenta as the midwife descended.

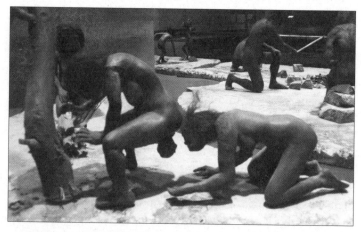

Figure 1: A museum display of human evolution in the Museo Nacional de Antropología, Mexico, shows an archaic woman semi-squatting with a midwife behind her. She doesn't appear to be using the handy tree, surely an oversight by the person who built the scene.

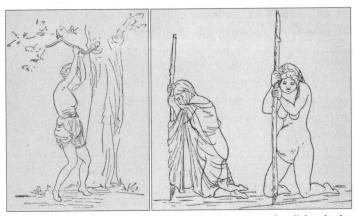

Figures 2 & 3: Using what is at hand to provide support for all four limbs (Engelmann, 1883).

(I wonder when humans stopped eating the placenta? I would hazard a guess that it was after we invented cooking and many of us developed a taboo against raw meat.)

Speculating on the origins of our own birth culture, during labour women would have carried on with their daily life, moving instinctively to find a comfortable position to cope with the contractions as they occurred. Women would have made use of what was readily at hand for support. Perhaps the first natural aid to labour was a tree; the women leant against it either facing forward or leaning back on it, or using a branch to support herself with her arms. A simple pole in the ground was used by some Native Americans according to Engelmann (1883).

The immediate proximity of the birth itself is signalled by pressure on the rectum and instinct may have led women to find a secluded spot and adopt the position that humans without the benefit of flush toilets adopt for defecation – squatting. At the hunter-gatherer phase of human existence any place away from the camp would have served the purpose. Women may or may not have called for help and other women may or may not have seen what was happening and followed to assist.

We have no way of knowing but, short of finding a nice safe tree for the birth, the rest of the monkey birth described above is likely to be similar to how our ancestors gave birth for, underneath our second skin of clothes, we are undoubtedly animals. Until the birth was imminent the early human first-time mother may not have realised what was happening to her but experienced mothers would have seen the signs and known that a baby was expected. It is likely that midwifery preceded language but with the advent of language came storytelling, sharing the accumulated wisdom of the band of humans, a sense of history, passing on culture to new generations. The birth story is one of the most compulsive tales there is to tell – I started writing my first book the day after the birth of my third child. Our current birth culture would tell you that both he and I were lucky to survive his birth – he was born at home – but we lived to tell the tale and it felt like the crowning experience of my life.

Hunter-gatherers had no need for furniture so we can start the story of the birth stool from the time when humans settled in one place, with the advent of agriculture, which first appeared about 12,000 years ago in the Middle East. Midwifery as a profession probably started around the same time. Sheila Kitzinger (2000) reports that the Inuit, a hunter-gatherer people who travelled in small bands, taught all their womenfolk basic midwifery skills – just in case they needed to help at a labour, but once people settled in one place in permanent homes the midwife could be easily located and sent for. For millennia midwives have helped women cope with labour and give birth in their own homes, from cave to cottage from tenement to palace. In ancient Egypt women are depicted giving birth on slightly raised platforms. The hieroglyphic symbol for birth depicts a raised up kneeling woman.

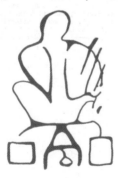

Figure 4: Egyptian hieroglyphic for birth. Woman seated on two stones. The three parallel lines represent suffering.

Again in Egypt we find documentary evidence for the use of two stones or a stool for birth. In the book of *Exodus* in the Bible relating to the Hebrew people's exile in Egypt, written perhaps 8,000 years ago, we find:

> The king of Egypt said to the Hebrew midwives, one of whom, was named Shiph'rah and the other Puah, 'When you serve as midwife to the Hebrew women, and see them upon the birth stool, if it is a son, you shall kill him; but if it is a daughter, she shall live.' But the midwives feared God, and did not do as the king of Egypt commanded them, but let the male children live.... So God dealt well with the midwives; and the people multiplied and grew very strong. (Exodus 1, 15-20 Revised Standard Version)

The words are actually spoken by an Egyptian, the king of Egypt. The Hebrew word was translated as 'birth stool' by the King James Version of the Bible, written between 1604 and 1611, but a more literal meaning is 'two stones'. The use of the word 'stool' in the translation implies that the woman is seated, but Engelmann (1883) has an illustration of a Persian woman kneeling forward on two piles of three bricks. I think this implies that women had a choice of position for birth. The Bible says 'see them upon the birth stool'. 'Upon' could mean either kneeling or sitting. If kneeling were the only position there would be no need for two stones spaced apart to allow for the passage of the baby.

Images and sculptures of women giving birth on stools go way back in time and are found on all sorts of artefacts ranging from wall decorations to vases, jugs, buckles and buildings. Usually they depict women in the act of giving birth – the second stage of labour. The woman is seated, leaning backwards into the arms of one or two people standing behind her and in front is a midwife preparing to receive the baby.

For four thousand years or more women used some type of birth stool or chair which was designed to lift her off the ground leaving just enough room for the baby to be born but allowing her to place her feet firmly on the ground. The birth stool or birth chair was invented over and over again. Throughout recorded history until the mid-1700s women are depicted as

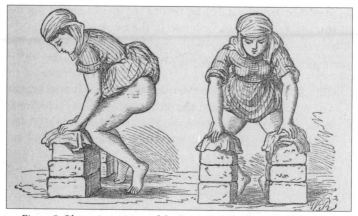

Figure 5: Obstetric position of the Persians (Engelmann, 1883).

using upright or semi-upright positions for birth, often with a birth supporter sitting behind them and the midwife seated in front ready to receive the baby. The first documentary evidence dates back thousands of years and takes the form of images depicting women giving birth. They are found on the walls of temples, carved in bas relief, on household objects such as vases and an ivory belt buckle or disguised as gargoyles hidden away out of sight on church roofs.

Birth was essentially women's business until the mid-eighteenth century. Ancient Greek and Latin texts had given instructions for midwives; medical intervention was restricted to cases of dire emergency, perhaps when brute force or instruments were needed to extract a dead infant, but doctors had no other professional interest in birth. As to the use of furniture, Aristotle (384-322 BC) wrote:

> As to the manner of the delivery, various midwives use different ways; some are delivered sitting on a midwife's stool. But, for my own part, I think that a pallet bed, girded, and placed near the fire, that the good woman may come on each side, and be the more readily assisted, is much the best way.

He goes on to describe the position universally favoured by doctors:

> … let the midwife lay the woman in a posture for delivery. ….

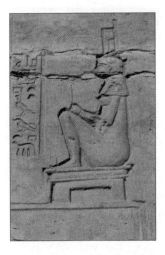

Figure 6: Temple on the Nile at Kom Obo. Egyptian woman giving birth seated on a special chair or stool.

Then let her lay the woman upon her back, having her head a little raised by the help of a pillow, having the like help to support her reins (loins) and buttocks, that her rump may lie high; for if she lie low she cannot very well be delivered. Then let her keep her knees and thighs as far asunder as she can, her legs being bowed towards her buttocks, and let her feet be stayed against a log or some other firm thing; and let two women hold her two shoulders, that she may strain out the birth with more advantage, holding in her breath, and forcing herself as much as possible, in like manner as when she goes to stool: for by such straining the diaphragm, or midriff, being strongly thrust downwards, necessarily forces down the womb, and the child in it.

Not being a Greek scholar, it is difficult to be certain, but the translation treats the woman as a passive object: 'let the midwife lay the woman... lay the woman upon her back ... having her head raised ... be delivered'. Aristotle's language betrays a medical attitude to complicated birth (his father was a doctor). This is all very well when birth is not straightforward but it presages the day when the doctor's attitude rubbed off on the midwife and changed her attitude to the women she cared for. It also foretells the development of the birth chair into the obstetric bed. The fundamental mistake in obstetrics has always been to assume that what is needed for abnormal birth is also needed for normal birth. The doctor's help and equipment is brought in before it is actually needed 'just in case'. The doctor's anticipated future requirements take precedence over the woman's current needs. This lack of perception of women's requirements for normal labour is sufficient in itself to change the course of the labour. The woman has less control over the positions she wants to adopt for her labour and, knowing that medical help is anticipated, she might already be losing faith in her ability to give birth. The anticipated need for intervention makes it more likely.

But it feels fundamentally unfair to blame Aristotle for the change of birth posture from an upright position to what Janet Balaskas and Sheila Kitzinger term the 'stranded beetle' position. For the next two thousand years or more the midwife was the person summoned for childbirth and she came, bringing with her the tool of her trade, the birth stool. (Following the custom of the day of naming actors by the tools of their trade, the playwright Ben Jonson, in his play *The Magnetic Lady*, named the midwife 'Mother Chair' after her profession – the heroine's niece had the somewhat bizarre name of Placentia Steel!)

Soranus of Ephesus (AD 98–138) has more to answer for than Aristotle; he seems to have been the first to advocate confining women to bed for labour. He advised that 'during labour a woman should be nursed in bed until delivery was imminent, and then moved to the birthing chair, when the midwife would sit opposite her, encouraging her to push' (Drife, 2002). His treatise, being written in Latin, escaped the attention of midwives but may have influenced the writings of early obstetricians who would know very little about the best

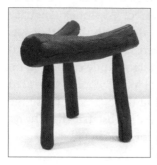

Figure 7: One has to admire the ingenuity of the carpenter who made this chair from a forked branch with three legs roughly inserted beneath. It is to be found in the Ceredigion Museum in Wales. The museum notes indicated that it has been used as a chopping block at some stage, which may account for its survival into the twenty-first century.

positions for early labour, being called in only towards the end if a woman was unable to deliver her baby by what is sometimes quaintly termed 'maternal effort'.

The first midwifery books were published soon after the dawn of the printed book. The first of these, Giovanni Savonarola's *Practica Maior* (Tract VI, Chapter XXI, rubric 32), was a textbook for doctors. It was written in Latin between 1440 and 1446 only ten years after the invention of moveable type which revolutionised the dissemination of knowledge. Savonarola describes the use of the birthing chair thus:

> First, the midwife ought to prepare a chair above which the parturient ought to stand, or rather, in relationship to which the parturient ought to position herself so as to make the birth quicker. And in diverse regions and cities women have diverse inventions, which are not possible for me to enumerate. But I should touch on their common [features] which are applicable in all cases.
>
> When she is finally in the act of giving birth, let the midwife order the pregnant woman to sit for the space of an hour or thereabouts. I say 'thereabouts' because there are some women so accustomed to giving birth that they give birth in one hour. For if it is not her first birth, the midwife ought to inform herself right from the start so that she knows how she ought to regulate herself vis-à-vis the pregnant woman. Then she should make her walk around, jumping sometimes on one foot, sometimes on the other, which is exceedingly helpful, or she should shout out forcefully, or she should hold her breath so that it presses on the lower parts. Likewise, she should have her hips rubbed and pressed in order to expel the foetus. And when the woman senses that the foetus is descending and the mouth of the womb is opening up with intensifying pains, and that the fluids begin to flow out in greater quantity, then let the midwife order that the pregnant woman sit upon the high seat with a cushion on its outer edge. And behind let [another] cushion be placed, and another woman to whom she can cling; or, if it is possible, let her stand on her own feet and let her suspend herself from the neck of a strong woman who holds her up. Or let her squat on her knees on a bed where she is supported by other women. And some

women, such as the Greeks, have a seat made in this manner, like this. [Presumably an illustration was meant to appear here, reproduced below from a translated edition.]

While the parturient sits upon the first semicircular outer edge [of the chair], behind her stands the [woman] who supports her, and she holds on to the cushion, and behind her is another woman slightly above her, holding and controlling her, on whom the woman leans for support. And this is a good method, although it is not used everywhere. But you can be certain, as I have heard tell from [women], no single procedure works [in all situations] because it is necessary to adapt according to the pains and the causes impeding the exit of the foetus.

The illustration on page 29 accompanies this text in later printed editions of the work. Talk of a 'high seat' is confusing; the seat is only 20 to 25 centimetres high. The text confirms that the seat was for the act of birth rather than for labour.

Monica Green considers that Savonarola's *Practica Maior* was the basis for a book written by Eucharius Rösslin in 1513, *The Rosegarden for Pregnant Women and Midwives*, but that he rewrote the section on birth chairs:

> In the lands of upper Germany and also in Italian regions the midwives have special chairs when the women are to give birth, and they are not high but cut out and hollow inside, as shown here. And they are to be made in such a manner that the woman is able to lean backwards with her back. The chair should be stuffed with cloths at the back, and when the time has come, the midwife is to reposition the cloths on the right or the left side as needed. And she is to sit before the woman, sedulously watching the movements of the child in the womb.

The Rosegarden became the standard midwifery textbook all over Europe and was translated into many languages. In England the 1545 edition, *The Byrth of Mankynde, Otherwyse Named the Woman's Booke* in 1545 further expanded the section on birth chairs:

> Then it will be meet for her to sit down leaning backward (in the

birth stool) in manner upright. For the which purpose in some regions (as in France and Germany) the midwives have stools for the purpose, which being not low, and not high from the ground be made so round wise and concave or hollow in the middle, that they may be received from underneath which is looked for [the baby] and the back of the stool leaning backward received the back of the woman, the fashion of which this stool, is set in the beginning of the birth figure hereafter. And when the time of labour is come, in the same stool ought to be put many clothes or rags in the back of it, that which the midwife may remove from one side to another according as necessity shall require. The midwife herself shall sit before the labouring woman and shall diligently observe and wait, how much, and after what means the child stirreth itself, also shall with her hands first anointed with the oil of almonds, or the oil of white lilies.

The 1545 edition also included recent anatomical drawings taken from Vesalius, the founder of modern anatomy. It remained in print for more than 100 years. Until the Renaissance, doctors

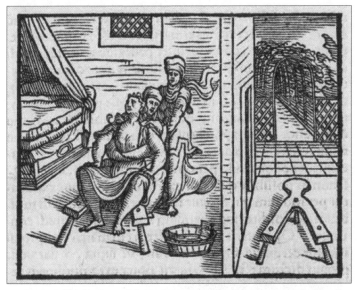

Figure 8: The birth stool Giovanni Savonarola illustrates in his book *Practica Maior*, a medical book published in 1550, demonstrates a continuity of form and function from the birth stool of Moses' time, but over the next four and a half centuries it changed out of all recognition.

had relied on classical works copied by hand in Greek or Latin but the advent of the printing press led to books being issued in translation and made accessible to more people. The process of translation demanded an attention to detail in choosing the right words in the vernacular tongue. The temptation to add one's personal opinion accounts for the gradually expanding sections on the birthing chair in the examples quoted above. Essentially we have a Greek text translated into Latin, then German then into English. The very act of translation itself may have fuelled a spirit of inquiry which was the springboard for the scientific advances in the Enlightenment; in the same way, the translation of the Bible into the vernacular led to the Reformation. Both the spirit of the Enlightenment and the Reformation were to play a part in paving the way for modern obstetrics. Doctors started to learn more about the anatomy of birth; theoretically, nature was something that could be understood scientifically and brought under man's control. This was the beginning of the transfer of power from church to professions. For the moment, however, the church still controlled midwives, which was deemed necessary because of their responsibility for bringing new souls into the world and

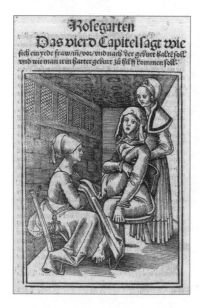

Figure 9: Title page from *The Rosegarden.*

baptising stillborn babies.

In France the church maintained its influence on birth by establishing a maternity section within the Hôtel Dieu, a Paris hospital, but the net result was to medicalise birth, firstly, by providing a training facility for doctors and midwives and, secondly, by disseminating the practice of using a special bed for delivery. The use of the horizontal position in labour and birth was reiterated by Ambroise Paré (1510–1590), barber-surgeon at the Hôtel Dieu in Paris, and by his successor, Jacques Guillemeau, who in 1609 wrote that it was 'for the women's comfort and to facilitate labour' (Dundes, 1987). Francois Mauriceau, a French obstetrician born in 1637, continued this French hospital tradition at the Hôtel Dieu and carried it over to births outside hospital, at the court of Louis XIV, who approved of the supine position because it enabled him to see his children being born.

The widespread adoption of the supine position for birth was perhaps the first instance of 'just in case' obstetrics which was to have such a profound influence on maternity care. To this day the horizontal position remains the standard position for labour and birth in the 'developed' world. Because the obstetrician needs to 'stand before' (Latin: *stet ob*) the woman to use his instruments, it was expedient for women to be confined to the bed:

> I studied this formerly in the Hôtel Dieu in Paris in a great number of accouchements which I did there. When the women which are to be delivered begin to be in labour, they go into a room which they call le chauffrey, where they are delivered on a small low bed, made specially for the purpose, and put before the fire; then as soon as they have been delivered, they go back to lie down on their own bed, which is frequently some distance away from the delivery room, where they walk very well on foot; which they could never do if their pubic bones, or those of the ilia were separated one from other. (Francois Mauriceau, 1668, *Traité des Maladies des Femmes Grosse*)

The very word accouchement contained the furniture for birth: an accoucheur was a man who led a woman to the childbirth couch. The idea of delivering in a bed is far more likely to have come from training doctors and midwives in the Paris hospital than Louis XIV's penchant for getting a better view of his mistress giving birth. Midwives trained for three months at the Hôtel Dieu:

> …with over a hundred confinements each month on an average, the four apprentice midwives at the hospital might expect to see three deliveries every day, which is almost one each, and in a busy three months each one could possibly have up to one hundred deliveries supervised by herself. This is very much more experience than any medical student in London today can possibly hope for in any of our teaching hospitals. It is not surprising that, with all this material and with the fame of its surgeons, any enterprising doctor in the seventeenth century who wished to study midwifery went to Paris… (Walter Radcliffe, 1947, *Milestones in Midwifery*)

In 1601 the Queen of France, Marie de Medici, grandmother of Louis XIV, had been attended by Louise Bourgeois (1563–1636), a midwife who wrote one of the first textbooks for midwives in 1609. Bourgeois did consider the needs of women in labour:

> A woman who wishes to keep about and can still do so until she is ready to give birth to the child, may be allowed to stand with legs apart, supported during the pains by two strong people, or she can have a low stool with a pillow on it, in front of a table, and can kneel on the pillow and put her arms on the table.

One hopes that her phrase 'allowed to stand' is a mistranslation; but perhaps even in 1609 women were losing control over their own labours and felt obliged to follow the instructions of their midwife rather than to follow their instincts. Sixty years later Mauriceau was describing the upright-leaning position, used by 'many in the country villages', as antiquated:

> …all women are not accustomed to be delivered in the same posture; some will be on their knees, as many in the country villages; others standing upright leaning with the elbows on a pillow upon a table, or on the side of a bed … but the best and

surest is to be delivered in their bed, to shun the inconvenience and trouble of being carried thither afterwards. (Mauriceau, *op cit*)

It is telling how Mauriceau contradicts himself – the luckless woman delivered in hospital had no trouble walking back to her hospital bed from the delivery room but it would be inconvenient for the woman employing a doctor in her own home who needed to be carried thither! One law for the paying patient, one for the charity case.

Mauriceau appears to have lifted his advice for women to give birth in a reclining position on a bed straight from Aristotle. The bed he describes is low, too low to allow easy access to the woman with instruments; moreover, his advice for women to deliver on a bed predates the use of obstetric forceps which had also originated in France, invented by the Chamberlen family, but forceps were not to be widely used for another seventy years. They had been demonstrated at the Hôtel Dieu but had been found wanting and the inventors emigrated to England, taking their forceps with them. In England it became fashionable to call in a man-midwife for birth and the second generation of the Chamberlen family also trained as doctors; the man-midwife had become a medical man and no man of standing could now allow his wife to give birth without a doctor in attendance. In the first half of the eighteenth century, after the death of the last in the line of Chamberlens, the secret of the forceps was revealed and they became the latest accessory for the fashionable doctor. If forceps were to be used, it was necessary to place the mother in a position where they could be used. Once the man-midwife had been replaced by the hospital-trained doctor, forceps had become respectable. But birth still took place in the home.

Attending women in childbirth was crucial for establishing a gentleman doctor in family practice which would give him a place in smart London society, but he needed to gain his credentials. The mid-eighteenth century saw the establishment of hospitals whose primary purpose was not to provide women with a safe place for birth, but to provide teaching material for young doctors. The first maternity hospital in London was the Lying-In Hospital for Married Women. It opened at the end of 1749 and it started training midwives two years later. It was followed in 1750 by the City of London Lying-In Hospital and the General Lying-In Hospital, founded in 1752. These hospitals were far from safe, quite the opposite; women died in their hundreds from puerperal fever. In 1828 the Lying-In Hospital for Married Women started sending out midwives to deliver patients in their own homes, perhaps because the death rate had become so high in hospital.

The industrial revolution saw large-scale migration from the countryside and as people moved to the towns they lost their country roots and their knowledge and respect for nature. They no longer kept a pig and hens in their back yards and lost familiarity with the natural processes of life and death. But the traditional midwife may have still brought her birthing stool with her.

Paid work was moving from home to factory. Dorothy Sayers (an Oxford don who wrote detective novels in her spare time) ascribes women's loss of power to the outsourcing of women's work from home to a separate workplace – spinning, weaving, dairying, brewing, all went to the factory (Sayers, 1938). Eventually birth itself was to be outsourced from the home. Before the industrial revolution, remunerative work at home could be combined with childcare, but once paid work was moved outside the home, women lost money, power and status. The industrial revolution was a disaster for working class women. Forced by poverty to go out to work, a woman could no longer breastfeed her baby and lost the contraceptive effect of lactation. Repeated childbearing and long working hours took their toll on the birth process itself. The state took an interest in maternity care only at the end of the nineteenth century when it found army recruits so weak and puny that it was hard to make a good soldier out of them (Tew, 1990).

Women were weakened physically because either they worked too hard or because they performed no physical labour at all. The status of a middle class man demanded that he had a wife who need not concern herself with physical labour, having servants to do all the heavy work. Perhaps childbearing really did become more difficult for a woman whose body was not used to physical work. It also became a question of status to call for the doctor rather than the midwife for birth. Birth became a distasteful unhealthy activity, for which the doctor was needed.

The story of birth since the industrial revolution is thus the tale of a clash of two cultures: the female midwifery culture based in the home which encouraged active birth in an upright posture, and the male obstetric culture based on techniques learned through practising on charity cases, powerless pauper women who had no one to champion them, lying on their hospital beds, giving up their babies at birth and often dying of puerperal fever carried on the hands and instruments of the men who attended them. Women giving birth in hospital were effectively little more than teaching material for doctors who would go on to deliver upper and middle class women at home for a fat fee.

There was money to be made from training midwives and gradually hospital-trained midwives were starting to compete with midwives who had learned their profession by apprenticeship. Hospital practices spilled over into the home. While the traditional midwives were no doubt still using birthing chairs, hospital-trained midwives were taught to deliver women on a bed. The old-fashioned birth chair had no place in hospital; moving a woman to an operating theatre when the time came to give birth was far easier. Operating theatres were places where the drama of birth was enacted with the obstetrician the central player and the woman reduced to an object on a table. These large rooms had benches arrayed in tiers and were designed for medical students to observe the use of obstetric instruments. Then as now there was money to be made from education. The role of hospitals in educating medical students increased the chance that professors would make the best of every teaching opportunity. Birth became a theatrical display.

Although doctors were trained in hospital, not all of them advocated using the bed throughout labour. In their perspective on maternal position in labour, Roberts and Méndez-Bauer (1980) point out that not all doctors put women to bed for labour. William Smellie (1752) commented on practice elsewhere:

In most all countries, the woman is allowed either to sit, walk about or rest on a bed until the uterine os is significantly dilated by the gravitation of the waters, or (when they are small in quantity) by the head of the foetus so that delivery is soon expected; then she is put in such a position as is judged most safe, easy and convenient for that purpose.

Merriman (1816) wrote that:

The patient may be allowed to sit, stand, kneel or walk about as her inclination may prompt her. If fatigued she should repose occasionally upon the bed or couch, but it is not expedient during these two stages that she should remain for a very long period of time in a recumbent posture.

These authors all observed that walking increased uterine activity because the cervix was stimulated by the weight of the fetus. As late as 1952 Williams was advising that 'a laboring woman should avoid too early recumbency' to prevent abnormal labour. Today's guidelines say similar things.

Rigby (1857), who was well aware of the social pressures that women laboured under, observed that a woman 'will in great measure, be guided by the arrangements which are made for her confinement and she will assume that position for which they are especially adapted'. This is as true today as it was 150 years ago. The arrangement of the birth furniture in every labour and delivery room today tells the woman what is expected of her and she complies with the instructions.

The story of the birth chair

The history of the transition from midwifery to obstetrics can be told through birth furniture. Midwives' chairs can be distinguished from doctors' chairs by the degree of craftsmanship displayed, whether or not there were leg extensions and whether or not the back could be lowered to place a woman in a horizontal position. It is fairly safe to assume that any folding chair was designed for use in the home and that the more elaborate and mechanical the chair, the more likely it was to have been designed and used by a medical man.

Amanda Carson Banks documents the changes in her book, *Birth Chairs, Midwives and Medicine* (1999). She travelled around Europe and the Americas, photographing birth chairs preserved in museums, measuring their dimensions and noting signs of missing parts. Some appear to have been purpose built, while others were adapted from household chairs.

Before medieval times chairs were not in general use in the home, and stools and benches were instead used for seating. Chairs tended to be used as a symbol of authority. Kings and priests would sit enthroned above the lower orders of mankind. Over time, the medieval midwife's stool, which could be carried in one hand in one piece, evolved into a birth chair. It acquired a back and the seat became higher until it reached the height of a household chair. The chair started to replace the stool in the home and birth chairs became more elaborate, having arms with handholds. As household chairs became more common they could be converted to birth chairs by the simple act of cutting out a hole in the seat.

Birth chairs started to reflect developments in furniture design. Having remained strictly utilitarian for thousands of years, fashion started to play a role, if only because the furniture makers who made them were learning new techniques such as joining panels with dowels and dovetailing joints. What is particularly striking about the surviving examples of birth chairs is that as time went by the height of the seat became higher and higher from the ground. Household chairs tend to be higher than stools, so the raised seat may have been a consequence of changing fashion in furniture, or it may simply have reflected women's changed habitual posture in everyday life and thus their preferred position for giving birth. The chairs now have hand holds and the more elaborate ones seem to have higher seats. It is likely that the higher the seat, the more hands-on care was probably given, whether by the midwife herself or a man-midwife called in for difficult cases. Amanda Banks shows a chair which has adjustable seat heights – 45, 55 and 65 centimetres. Even the lowest height is nearly double the height of the earliest stools. When instead of merely receiving the baby, midwives began to subject women to 'tugging and stretching' (Donnison, 1977) they needed to consider their own posture, and to be able to see what they were doing.

The birth chair was too deeply embedded in female culture to be lost altogether and birth still took place at home but the birth chair now underwent modifications to cater for the doctor, should he be called for. The seat became even higher, so high that the mother could no longer brace herself against the ground and now foot supports were necessary. When it became customary to call for the doctor for all middle class births regardless of need, the doctor would bring his own chair, designed to place women in a suitable position for obstetric instruments to be used. As time passed chairs became ever more elaborate; the male passion for gadgetry and technology was made manifest in the birth chair. The design became much more elaborate, reflecting the fees the doctor would charge. Eventually it became a chair that could be turned into a table, by lowering the back of the chair and raising the woman's legs on stretchers.

From a chair that could be turned into a table it was only a short step to turn the table into a bed. Obstetric tables and obstetric beds were designed for use in hospital for the benefit of doctors. The birth chair became more complicated when doctors started to take over birth in the home. From this it was but a short step to the obstetric table. Today no labour ward delivery room is without one.

In my quest to design a piece of furniture to enable women to labour more comfortably, I spent hours on Google images, looking and looking. One search term I entered was 'nursing chair' and having always assumed that these bedroom

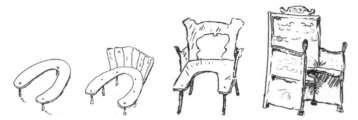

Figure 10: From stool to chair ...

chairs were for 'nursing' i.e. for breastfeeding mothers, it finally dawned upon me that 'nursing' might perhaps mean 'midwifery'. Hospital-trained midwives were proud of their training and preferred to be known as 'nurse' leaving the term 'midwife' for those with no formal training. (I was born with the help of Nurse Austin, who also delivered my sisters and half brother.) Some of these nursing chairs may have been designed for labour rather than breastfeeding. A chair without arms is not always ideal for breastfeeding but a low chair with a wide and deep base is very useful for kneeling in labour. Such a chair will accommodate the full length of the leg below the knee, it is near the ground, and it is wide enough for a woman to be able to shift her weight about. The chairs often had a high back with a scroll at the top for her to lean on. The small side arms of some of these chairs may have served to add strength against the unusual forces generated by women leaning against the back of a chair, they may have provided a sense of containment for a labouring woman or if a little larger they may have been used for hand holds.

Hospital-trained midwives would have attended middle class women who had both the space and the money to purchase such a chair for the bedroom, but it would have been 'indelicate' for its purpose to be immediately apparent – the chairs lacked a cut out section for upright birth. Searching online for *'prie dieu'* also brought up pictures of nursing chairs. A *prie dieu* is purpose designed for kneeling to pray. Could some nursing chairs have been designed for kneeling in labour? If they were, it was the last time for 100 years that anyone would consider the needs of women for physical support in labour.

By the beginning of the twentieth century the birthing

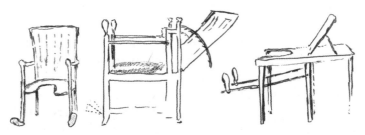

Figure 11: ... and from chair to table.

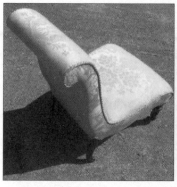 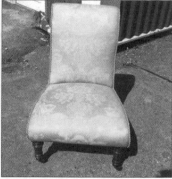

Figure 12: Known as a 'nursing chair' was this bedroom chair actually designed for labour?

chair was all but forgotten; all that remained was a horseshoe-shaped hole two thirds of the way down from the head of the obstetric bed, and the leg extensions had been raised above the height of the birthing platform to become stirrups. Straps had been added to tie women in place, immobilising them completely. The woman had been rendered a passive recipient of medical attention. Women were confined to bed in hospital to give birth for three generations. Birth went on at home much as it had done before but without the help of a chair or stool.

The birth chair didn't emerge again until the 1970s. The 1960s had ushered in electronic fetal monitoring (EFM), also known as cardiotocography (CTG); artificial oxytocin could be given by drip feed and used to induce labour or speed it up; prostaglandins could be used to induce labour. Such interventions made labour more painful and epidural anaesthesia was not yet widely used. Women started to lobby for better care. The Society for the Prevention of Cruelty to Pregnant Women was founded, later renaming itself as the Association for Improvements in the Maternity Services (AIMS), and is still active today because it is still needed. Germaine Greer's *The Female Eunuch* was published in 1970; women wanted to reclaim ownership of their own bodies. Ina May Gaskin's caravan of hippy buses end up in Tennessee and the colony was teaching itself midwifery by trial and error with a little help from a doctor who still attended home births; Ina May's book, *Spiritual Midwifery*, was first published in 1977 and has remained in print ever since. In the 1980s a 'Stand and Deliver' rally was held on Hampstead Heath in London; women were protesting against the forced birthing positions mandated by obstetricians at the Royal Free Hospital (Balaskas, 1983). Women were starting to rebel against medicalised childbirth and the alternative birth movement started.

Birth chairs reappeared in the 1980s. There was an expensive birthing chair for hospitals costing $5,400 in 1981 and available in 400 hospitals around North America – according to a report in an *Ottawa Citizen* newspaper. Until reading further round the subject, I had assumed that the hospital birth chair was made available in an attempt to make hospital birth more consumer friendly, to compete with birth centres which had started to offer an alternative to American women, but the Century Birthing Chair was actively promoted by Roberto Caldeyro-Barcia, a physiologist and obstetrician who had been interested in labour and birth positions since the 1950s, when he was investigating the effect of posture on the progress of labour. The EZ Birthing Chair was illustrated in a medical journal (Reid and Harris, 1988) in a paper on alternative birth positions attempting to change doctors' view on birth position.

The wedge-shaped Kitzinger cushion and the Gardosi cushion were also designed for hospital use to allow a woman to give birth in a sitting position on the bed while taking pressure off her tailbone. The Gardosi cushion was designed by a doctor and had the luxury of being subjected to clinical trials, which showed a beneficial effect. Both of these could be used in obstetric units.

In the USA birthing centres and midwives adopted a low-tech answer to birthing position, getting local handymen to make them birth stools and chairs.

Over the last 30 years there have been various attempts to enable women to adopt different positions for labour and birth. The Association of Radical Midwives even designed a squatting bar to attach to an obstetric bed. I gave birth to my first child in an obstetric chair which was situated in a separate delivery room, which also contained an obstetric delivery couch. Since then the fashion has been to have just one room for labour and birth, and most rooms have state-of-the-art obstetric beds. If a trip to the operating theatre proves necessary, the bed doubles up as a trolley. Some obstetric beds can convert into birth chairs. While obstetric beds can be manipulated to assume different heights and positions, the cleaners may have left them set flat with an incontinence pad neatly placed ready for the first vaginal examination. The environment is clinical and stark to reduce the risks of infection – everything must be able to be steam cleaned. Around the bed is all the paraphernalia of modern technological birth: a fetal monitoring machine and drip stand are alongside, on the wall behind there is a panel with lines and tubes for this and that – piped in gas and air, and oxygen, a monitoring BP, pulse oximetry, temperature – whatever modern medicine thinks is necessary for safe birth. There is a desk and chair for the midwife to use for the endless record-keeping required and a bedside chair for the partner. Depending on the hospital culture, other equipment may be already at hand – birth balls (large gym balls), beanbags and mats may be in the room already – or it may be tidied away in a store room. A quick question on Facebook while trying to catch up with modern hospital practice showed that furniture in the birth room is fairly adaptable but that how it is used depends on women's expectations and midwives' comfort in working with women in different positions. Most hospitals now have one or two labour rooms with birth pools but they can only be used if a midwife trained in water birth is available and willing. Some midwives may lack the confidence to care for women using birth pools and some may have back problems which preclude caring for women labouring in water.

It is ironic that birth centres run by midwives for low-risk women have a far greater variety of equipment available to help women find different positions for labour and birth. Some have even hidden the bed away, taking away the temptation to use it. The Bradbury couch, made of vinyl-covered foam, is a bed-shaped couch with a semi-circular hole cut out of it

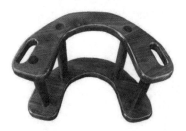

Figure 13: A modern homely birthing stool.

half way along one side and is designed to allow women to make use of the floor. There is a birth pool in nearly every room; there are sofas, couches and rocking chairs, birth stools with or without backs, slings, ropes to pull on and even wall bars which, when combined with birth balls, offer an even larger range of positions for the mother, her midwife and her birthing partner. Women labelled as high risk need these things too. They need a less forbidding, kinder environment and a midwife who will enable them to feel relaxed enough to let go of their preconceptions about how birth should be and, as Ina May Gaskin says: 'Let their monkey do it'.

Conclusion

Thus the bed still dominates the delivery room and the default position for labour and birth is horizontal; all other positions are labelled 'alternative'. Delivery rooms in modern hospitals are still designed around the bed; although most large maternity units do now have one or two birth pool rooms. Even today only low-risk women are routinely allowed the option of alternative birth positions; routine electronic monitoring of high-risk women usually requires a woman to have her movement constricted by the length of the leads connecting her to a CTG machine. Birth centres provide an environment more conducive to freedom of movement for labouring women but are open only to low-risk women.

When maternity care was finally subjected to scientific scrutiny, vertical positions were tested as the 'new' treatments against the long-time standard horizontal care. At the same time, paradoxically, upright positions tended to be seen as old

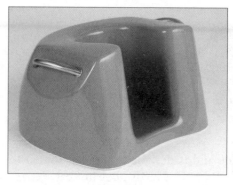

Figure 14: A modern stool designed to pass health and safety checks.

fashioned; a paper by a Canadian doctor (Reynolds, 1991) is entitled 'Primitive delivery positions in modern obstetrics'. Would modern obstetrics ever be able to incorporate upright positions? The jury is still out. So what is the evidence?

3 Research evidence

Inquiry into the purpose for which any of the various positions which women have from time to time assumed while in labor, will show that the choice has been made more from the force of custom, from caprice, ignorance and from a blind submission to authority – exercised by those who make unwarrantable pretensions to skill in midwifery, than from knowledge deduced from facts gained by careful study and close observation. (A P Clarke, US obstetrician, *Journal of the American Medical Association* 1891; **16**: 433.)

The last chapter showed how positions for birth came to be dictated by force of custom and blind submission to authority, the authority of medical men who preferred their patients to be on the bed. Doctors claimed their authority from science but for the most part obstetrics remained a skilled manual occupation with its practitioners relying on the use of instruments to perform surgical procedures when they considered them necessary. The management of labour was largely based on obstetric opinion but, eventually, scientific research was carried out. There are three types of scientific knowledge recognised by obstetrics: clinical trials – testing interventions on patients; epidemiology – the study of the patterns, causes, and effects of health and disease conditions in defined populations; and anatomy and physiology – how the body functions. Evidence from physiology does not appear to figure highly in the obstetric mindset. Despite theoretical knowledge of the increased mobility of the pelvis during pregnancy, which increases the available space in the pelvis, obstetricians actually hardly ever see this because most procedures are performed with the woman on her back. The only exception is when performing manoeuvres for shoulder dystocia, where one of the baby's shoulders gets trapped at the top of the pelvic inlet; manoeuvres usually involve passively moving the woman's legs or, more recently, turning her on to the all-fours position.

Uterine contractions have been found to be more efficient in the sitting position increasing uterine pressure by improving the alignment of the fetus to the cervix (Chen *et al*, 1987). Blood supply to the mother's uterus and the placenta is restricted in the supine position because the weight of the uterus is constricting the blood vessels which leads to aortocaval compression. The abdominal aorta and the inferior vena cava which lie in front of the spine are compressed by the uterus when a pregnant woman lies on her back, leading to low maternal blood pressure and a 20% drop in blood flow. This can be mitigated by turning a woman on to her side, tilting her as much as 34 degrees to the left lateral position. It probably reveals the extent of obstetric knowledge that this information came from a paper headed by an anaesthetist (Kinsella, Whitwam and Spencer, 1992). The authors state that 10% of women show signs of aortocaval compression, some even when in the standing or semi-recumbent positions. Johnstone *et al* (1987) found a decrease in fetal oxygenation associated with the supine position when comparing it to a side-tilted position. Supine positions during second stage have also been found to result in more frequent abnormal fetal heart rate patterns (Marttila *et al*, 1983).

Even evidence from physiology as compelling as this comes at the very bottom of the ratings list for the quality of clinical evidence. The National Institute for Care and Health Excellence (NICE is the body that produces the guidelines on how to manage birth in England and Wales) includes evidence from physiology only as part of expert opinion. I find it extraordinary that there is so little interest in the physiology of birth and will devote the next five chapters to it in an attempt to redress the balance a little. Nevertheless, research into physiology has had a large effect on the management of birth, largely because of the vested interests of drug and technology companies. Technologies such as electronic fetal monitoring (EFM), also known as cardiotocography (CTG), which were originally developed to study normal physiology, were seized upon with alacrity by obstetricians for clinical use. There was a similar swift reaction to physiological research into the hormones of labour. Almost as soon as physiologists had synthesised a hormone known to be involved in labour, the obstetricians would start experimenting with it clinically – largely a process of trial and error. Trial and error eventually gave way to randomised controlled trials (see below) and these are now claimed to give a scientific basis to obstetric treatment, but the physiology underlying the treatment tends to be poorly understood, disregarded, unknown or forgotten.

Physiologists are interested in normal birth but for obstetricians normal birth is an outcome, not a process to be studied. Clinical practice may change if there is unassailable evidence of better outcomes with a new form of treatment and hospital guidelines also encourage its use – even then it is an uphill struggle unless powerful people have a vested interest in changing practice. Hospital guidelines are written by a team headed by an obstetrician whose training has been biased towards curing the abnormal. In the case of position in labour, the bed and the supine position have been firmly established as the norm for the last 200 years and there are centuries of obstetric opinion to overcome and, added to that, half a century of anaesthetist involvement in birth.

Observational study

Carlson *et al* (1986) attempted to find out what positions women choose to adopt during labour in hospital when left to their own devices. They observed 80 women in spontaneous labour, coding their position at 15-30 minute intervals in very early labour and 5-15 minute intervals during active labour and second stage. What is perhaps most enlightening is that their codes did not include supine lying at all – presumably because they did not see it. They observed women lying on their left or right sides, sitting in bed at 45°, upright in bed at 90°, walking, squatting, sitting in a rocking chair or sitting upright in a chair. They found that women tended to assume a larger number of different positions in early labour (average three), fewer positions in the active phase (average two), one position in the deceleration phase (known as transition in the

UK), and one for second stage. Five positions accounted for all but 6.9% of observations. These were the two side-lying positions on the bed and sitting on the bed at 45° or 90°, and walking. The women chose an average of 7.5 positions throughout labour, which the authors attribute to women's desire for mobility and change. They concluded that it would be: '… appropriate to help support patients in their desire to vary their positions in labour. This can be facilitated by birthing chairs or beds to accommodate any maternal position and to aid in changing positions.'

The authors pointed out that they were unable to observe what positions women adopted before coming into hospital. They were aware that choices of position would be constrained by available furniture. It would be useful to repeat the exercise for women giving birth at home. This observational study is particularly useful because it recognises that women are not static, particularly in the early stages of labour. They do not decide on one position and stick to it, although the authors did find that the further advanced in labour, the fewer positions were chosen.

There are so many different aspects to maternal position in labour that it is difficult to research it as a whole. The distinction is usually between an upright position or not and first or second stage of labour. Earlier studies never looked at the second stage of labour since hospital practice almost always required women to be lying on their side or on their back. A fairly recent study escapes inclusion in review articles because it compares two different upright positions in the second stage of labour. Ragnar *et al* (2006) compared sitting and kneeling during the second stage of labour, which are both classified as upright positions, and found that there was no significant difference in length of labour, but the kneeling position was associated with a more favourable maternal experience and less pain compared with the sitting position.

Advantages of the upright position

Comfort, pain and length of labour

Asking women to mark their pain on a visual analogue scale, Adachi *et al* (2003) studied 58 women who alternated between sitting and supine at 15-minute intervals between 6 and 8 centimetres of dilatation. They found that pain scores for the sitting position were significantly lower than those for the supine position. This held for women experiencing continuous lumbar pain as well as those feeling pain only during contractions. Méndez-Bauer *et al* (1975) also chose an experimental design where women acted as their own controls. This time they alternated between lying and standing. Nineteen out of the 20 women were more comfortable in the standing position and fifteen reported less pain despite stronger contractions.

A review by Lupe and Gross in 1986 found that many investigators have reported that mobility in labour results in greater maternal comfort and ability to tolerate labour, and decreased use of anaesthesia and analgesia. Bloom *et al* (1998) found no clinical differences between walking in labour or not, but it is perhaps significant that 99% of women in the walking group said they would choose to walk again in labour. In her study of ambulation in labour, Flynn (1978) found a significantly reduced need for analgesia in women who walked during labour. Andrews and Chrzanowski (1990) found that women randomised to an upright rather than a recumbent position had significantly shorter labours (from 4-10 cm) but reported no difference in comfort levels, although presumably women were in discomfort for a shorter length of time.

Clinical trials

Evidence from clinical trials takes precedence over evidence from basic physiological science. Experienced midwives might attempt to prevent or ameliorate a slow labour using their knowledge of the physiology and mechanisms of labour; however, inexperienced midwives may call for obstetric assistance sooner rather than later. In any case, hospital guidelines require midwives to call a doctor for such eventualities as a slower than average rate of cervical dilatation. The guidelines are written using the evidence of clinical trials which are designed to ascertain the most effective form of intervention. Clinical trials try to take individuals – the individual woman, the individual midwife and the individual doctor – out of the picture altogether. They attempt to find out what treatment works best for most women most of the time. It is difficult to reconcile the concept of woman-centred care, offering women informed choice of treatment, with the reality of management by protocols and algorithms (flow charts specifying treatment pathways) designed around clinical trials.

Clinical evidence is a numbers game – the larger the numbers involved, the more convincing the evidence is said to be. It is therefore surprising that no use is made of the epidemiological evidence hidden within the routinely collected NHS Maternity Statistics for England (HSCIC, 2013). This rich source of whole population statistics on hospital procedures could answer many questions about the safety of obstetric interventions and I cannot understand why it is not used for this purpose, although one problem is that outcomes for the baby are not linked to the outcomes for the mother so vast swathes of potentially valuable information are lost. Clinical audit is also a valuable tool in evaluating the effectiveness of treatment in individual hospitals, most of which have thousands of births each year, but this evidence is deemed less trustworthy than the results of clinical trials.

Randomised controlled trials

The randomised controlled trial (RCT) is now considered the best form of clinical evidence because it attempts to give an impartial answer to a clinical question where there is genuine doubt or controversy. In order to avoid unconscious bias on the part of the researcher or caregivers, patients are assigned at random to one of two groups, one group receiving the treatment under trial and the other receiving a different treatment (positive control group) or no treatment (placebo control group). Large numbers of clinical trials all looking at similar interventions can be grouped together and their results combined to form a systematic review, the very highest rated form of evidence. The evidence itself usually concerns the risks and benefits of performing a specific clinical intervention over not intervening.

Clinical research is an academic discipline usually conducted in hospitals attached to universities. Research rarely takes place in any place other than a hospital. Apart from studies of place of birth itself, women labouring at home are not included in research trials. Women choosing home birth are deemed to be too much of a special self-selected group and not typical of the childbearing population as a whole but they are in fact the women most likely to experience normal labour. The research agenda is set by those with power – doctors and hospitals – and those with money – drug and technology companies. Research by midwives into normal birth didn't really take off until midwifery education moved into the universities in the 1990s.

In the late 1980s RCTs of upright position were usually related to novel obstetric chairs (Stewart and Spiby, 1989; Crowley et al, 1991), while more recent research on maternal position relates to low-dose 'walking' epidurals (COMET Study Group, 2001). Hospitals supply a steady stream of experimental subjects; it's so much easier to conduct research on captive patients who are confined to one place. Women labouring in hospitals can be found on or near a bed in the labour ward. While, theoretically, it would be possible to do RCTs in birth centres, the notion of randomising women to one 'treatment' or another is in direct conflict with the concept of individualised, woman-centred care, which birth centres do their best to provide. When an RCT involving a birth centre is performed it concerns outcomes for birth centre care itself. RCTs in perinatal care (care provided during labour and birth) can only really take place in an environment where women are already placed under the social restraints inherent in institutional care. Trial protocols specifically try to vary only one aspect of treatment at a time so that results will reflect the parameter which has been changed and nothing else. Only women with little control over their care will be willing to be randomised to one group or another.

Chan's 1963 study of 200 first-time mothers was one of the earliest to study upright position for labour. He found no advantage to an upright position in first and second stage of labour. However, the upright group in this study consisted of women who remained on the bed propped up with a bed-rest at an angle of 45°-60°, and it is arguable whether this should be regarded as an upright position (Coppen, 2005). One purpose of his study was to investigate whether it was indeed practicable even to maintain an erect posture during labour and delivery: 'Some patients, when they were not under constant supervision, tended to slip lower and lower down the bed-rest and were eventually found to lie curled or doubled up near the end of the bed. Eight patients did in fact complain quite bitterly of the erect position.' The propped up position was found to be awkward by the obstetrician in most of the cases and was said to be responsible for 'a great deal of inconvenience in seven instances'. The difficulties experienced by the women were attributed to the use of bed-rests. Chan wondered whether the design of the bed was to blame and suggested using 'cardiac or surgical' beds which had head ends which could be raised: 'The cost of such beds, however, may be considerable; and unless the erect position can be convincingly proved to be definitely advantageous such expenditure will not prove worth while.' (The money has since been found. Today most labour rooms contain an obstetric bed costing as much as £8,000.)

Fetal monitoring in the upright position

Continuous fetal monitoring is monitoring by machine, the leads of which tethered women to a fixed place, usually a bed. This worried a doctor, Anna Flynn, who was concerned that one of the major causes of maternal death, thromboembolism (blood clots) was associated with prolonged bed rest. In 1976 she and her colleague tested a device on 30 'ambulant patients in labour' which used fetal scalp electrodes to monitor the fetal heart via radiotelemetry (Flynn and Kelly, 1976). Eighteen of the women were expected to give birth without problem and 12 were deemed to be 'at risk'. Three of the women had induced labours. Women were 'returned to bed' for the delivery. Results of this initial testing of the device were good, with 28 normal births and two women needing forceps. All infants were born in good condition, with Apgar scores (marks out of 10 for the baby's condition recorded at one minute and five minutes after birth) averaging 8.87 at one minute and 9.93 at five minutes. Two years later Flynn and Kelly had added contraction monitoring to the telemetry device and performed a randomised controlled trial of 68 women (Flynn *et al* 1978). They found labour to be significantly shorter with ambulatory monitoring, women needed less analgesia and there were fewer fetal heart abnormalities. They recommended that 'The advantages to the mother and her fetus indicate that ambulation in labour should be encouraged....'

Upright position as a treatment for prolonged labour

In a 1987 letter to the *British Medical Journal*, Geoffrey Chamberlain, who was later to become President of the Royal College of Obstetricians and Gynaecologists, advocated walking in labour, declaring that:'

The supine position should be avoided at any stage of labour. The hazards of supine hypotension, particularly among those women receiving epidural anaesthesia, are well documented. Further, both Turnbull and Caldeyro-Barcia *et al* have claimed that the lateral position is better for uterine action than the supine position. Several groups have claimed that standing and walking not only shorten labour but also ease the discomfort of the mother. Labour in the vertical position, on the other hand, is associated with increases in contraction intensity but not with contraction frequency, increases in total uterine activity, and higher resting intrauterine pressures. Read *et al* have suggested that the upright posture may be as effective as oxytocin for augmenting an inefficient labour.

Read's study (1981) was very small but very interesting. Fourteen women who failed to progress in the active phase of labour, and who required augmentation for 'inadequate' contractions were randomised into ambulation (8) or oxytocin (6). Was this the first time that 'ambulation' was deemed a 'treatment'? Internal fetal monitoring was used in all patients for a 30-minute baseline reading and two-hour study periods, with telemetry used in the women who walked. The study looked at changes in cervical dilation, contraction frequency, intensity, the baseline tone of the uterus and uterine activity. Labour progress was slightly but not significantly better in the ambulatory group. There was an immediate increase in uterine activity in the ambulatory group. The authors concluded: 'These initial observations seem to indicate that, in terms of labour progress and initial effects on uterine activity, ambulation is as effective as oxytocin for the enhancement of labour and warrants further investigation.'

Hemminki and his colleagues did investigate further in 1985 with a randomised controlled trial of 57 women; 60% of those in the ambulant group delivered their babies without oxytocin and, on average, had a shorter second stage of labour. The women themselves had relatively positive views of their experiences. In the oxytocin group, on the other hand, the women suffered from stronger contractions before pushing, and some had 'excessively strong contractions'. The trial was too small to judge which treatment was better for the infant's health. 'Nevertheless, the women's opinions and the quality of their contractions demonstrate that more attention should be paid to ambulation as a treatment for protracted labour.'

If an upright posture can indeed prevent the use of oxytocin to augment labour, there may be far-reaching beneficial consequences. In his book, *Childbirth and the Future of Homo Sapiens* (2013), another doctor, Michel Odent, is eloquent on the dangers of overuse of artificial oxytocin in labour because it is thought to disrupt the hormonal system which has evolved to bond mother and child.

Evidence-based obstetrics

Obstetricians were renowned for variations in their preferred management of birth. Midwives used to have to check the notes to see which obstetrician a woman was booked under to find out how he liked 'his patients' to be managed, for example, whether the woman should have continuous fetal monitoring or an episiotomy, whether she was 'allowed' to eat or drink. Guidelines are supposed to put a stop to this variation (Schram, 2013). It is not really so surprising that management of labour varied so widely between consultants. In most other areas of hospital medicine, patients are admitted to hospital because their bodies are malfunctioning, and treatment addresses the specific malfunction, but obstetrics concerns itself with healthy 'patients' whose bodies are performing a natural function. Whether or not to interfere with a natural function is a question of defining what is normal and what is abnormal. If normal, then watchful waiting might be the preferred option, if abnormal, then medical treatment may be considered necessary. Obstetric opinion still varies enormously. The amount of intervention depends on how much trust obstetricians place in women and their bodies, their confidence in midwives to spot deviations from normal, and how much power and control they wish to have over both women and midwives.

Archie Cochrane was the pioneer of evidence-based medicine, believing that treatment should be based on evidence not medical opinion. He awarded obstetrics the wooden spoon for having the worst evidence base to its interventions:

> The specialty missed its first opportunity in the sixties when it failed to randomise the confinement of low-risk pregnant women at home or in hospital. Then having filled the emptying beds by getting nearly all pregnant women into hospital, the obstetricians started to introduce a whole series of expensive innovations into the routines of pre- and post-natal care and delivery, without any rigorous evaluation. The list is long but the most important were induction, ultrasound, fetal monitoring and placental function tests. (Cochrane 1979)

What a pity that all those emptying beds had to be filled; one of the most radical changes in obstetric care which was never tested at all had been the introduction of the hospital bed itself in Paris 300 years before. If a bed was all that was provided for labouring women, then they would be forced to use it. Labour and delivery on the bed was the default maternal position for practically all research into obstetric treatment that wasn't related to position in labour, but it seems that the bed itself has never been subjected to clinical trials.

Cochrane proposed that treatment based purely on medical opinion (or preference) should be replaced by treatment based on clinical research evidence obtained through RCTs. Some RCTs had already been performed. The Oxford Database of Perinatal Trials was set up in 1986 to 'foster cooperative and coordinated research in the field of childbirth' (Chalmers *et al*, 1986) and it started to collate the results of clinical trials into the same or similar treatment and analyse them in meta-analyses which, by increasing the numbers, gives increased statistical power to detect real differences between the two treatments. The database led to the publication in 1990 of *Effective Care in Pregnancy and Childbirth* (Chalmers *et al*), a two-volume work of 1,300 pages based on 3,000 clinical research studies into the evidence for routine procedures during childbirth. These were divided into four categories, forms of care reducing negative outcomes, those that were promising but needed further evaluation, care with unknown effects, and forms of care that should be abandoned in the light of available evidence. In 1990 there emerged a long list of accepted practices and beliefs that should be abandoned, including the recommendation that all women should give birth in hospital. Paperback guides to the main work were published. In the 1989 *Guide to Effective Care in Pregnancy and Childbirth* (Enkin *et al*, 1989) position in the first stage merited its own section but by the third (and last) edition (Enkin *et al*, 2000) maternal position for the first stage of labour was considered only as it pertained to the birth environment. Women allocated to groups where they laboured and gave birth in 'home-like' settings used less pain medication on average and were slightly less likely to have their labour augmented by artificial oxytocin. The authors suggested that 'If renovations are desired they should be targeted towards factors that would encourage changes in behavior, such as removing lithotomy poles and replacing uncomfortable delivery beds with comfortable furniture and cushions.' Perhaps the authors thought that the argument for freedom of movement in active labour had already been won? The third edition did, however, consider position for the second stage: 'Constraining women to adopt positions that they find awkward or uncomfortable can only be justified if there is good evidence that the policy has important advantages for the health of either the mother or her baby.'

Clinical trials reviewed in the *Guide to Effective Care in Pregnancy and Childbirth*, or ECPC, as the book came to be known, showed that with upright postures the second stage was shorter and episodes of severe pain less frequent. Trials of birth chairs or stools showed fewer episiotomies (cutting the perineum, the birth outlet) but more second-degree tears. There was an increased tendency to postpartum haemorrhage which the authors attributed to perineal trauma and obstructed venous return. These disadvantages were offset by fewer abnormal fetal heart rate patterns. Some birth attendants reported inconvenience but there was a consistently positive response from the women who used an upright position for birth. The overall conclusion was that: 'Women should be encouraged to give birth in the position they find most comfortable, with the exception that the untilted supine position should be avoided.' (Enkin *et al*, 2000)

Cochrane reviews

Following the success of the obstetric database set up on the advice of Archie Cochrane, the Cochrane Collaboration was established in 1993 and carried on the work of producing systematic reviews of evidence, extending this beyond maternity care to other areas of medical care. Cochrane reviews are considered the gold standard in evidence-based care but they are designed to compare intervention with no intervention and thus exclude research which is designed merely to observe normal physiology, which is still sadly lacking in the literature and which is so hard to observe in the hospital environment. Nevertheless, there is a fair amount of research on position in labour and birth contained in Cochrane reviews.

The latest Cochrane review of mother's position in the first stage of labour (Lawrence *et al*, 2013) is a meta-analysis of 25 studies, involving 5,218 women, and comes out firmly in favour of the upright position and mobility. Labour is about one hour 20 minutes shorter; there is a reduction in caesarean birth, less use of epidural anaesthesia and fewer babies admitted to special care:

> There is little doubt that women should be encouraged to utilise positions which give them the greatest comfort, control and benefit during first stage labour. As women in most western societies now lie in bed for the entire duration of their labour, it is important that they understand the risks and benefits of the positions they choose.... women should be encouraged and supported to use upright and mobile positions of their choice during first stage labour, as this may enhance the progress of their labour and may lead to better outcomes for themselves and their babies. (Lawrence *et al*, 2013)

The Cochrane review into position in second stage for women labouring without an epidural (22 studies, 7,280 women) also shows that the scientific evidence favours the upright position, reducing the risk of surgical intervention with forceps delivery and episiotomy:

> Women should be encouraged to give birth in comfortable positions, which are usually upright.
> The review of trials found the studies were not of good quality, but they showed that when women gave birth on their backs there was more chance for an assisted delivery, e.g. forceps, there was a higher chance of requiring cuts to the birth outlet, but there was less blood loss. More research is needed. (Gupta, 2012)

Research into the upright position for second stage when a woman has epidural anaesthesia has not led to clear-cut conclusions:

The five randomised controlled trials (involving 879 women) evaluated in this review do not show a clear effect of any upright position compared with a lying down position. The trials are small however and cannot rule out any small important benefits or harms, so women should be encouraged to take up the position they prefer. (Kemp *et al*, 2013)

The bed

The trial I would like to see for position in labour has never been done. All trials have taken place in hospitals where, by the force of custom alone, every room contains a bed. This alone raises everyone's expectations that women should use the bed for labour. It is hard to see why there ever was a need to confine women to bed for the first stage of labour. An examination couch was all that was necessary for the doctor; while the cervix was still opening up there was little for him to do. The woman needed to be supine only for vaginal examination, to see how far on in labour she was, for palpation of the abdomen to determine how the fetus was lying in the uterus, and for amniotomy, breaking the waters, the most common surgical procedure in the first stage of labour. But the bed was such a standard piece of hospital equipment that it would have been unthinkable not to have one and once there it has proved impossible to dislodge. Fetal monitoring equipment was designed around a passive woman lying in a bed. Now that fetal monitoring by telemetry is more widely available, it would be easy to perform a clinical trial of women labouring with a bed in the room and women labouring with a hard examination couch and other furniture but no bed in the room but, to my knowledge, this has never been done. This would be a true test of freedom of movement. Of course a woman should also be able to request a bed.

Ellen Hodnett, a Canadian midwife, conducted a pilot study in 2009 and modified a labour room to remove the standard hospital bed, adding equipment to promote an ambience of relaxation, mobility, and calm. Sixty-two women were randomised to a standard room or the 'ambient' room. She found that 19 women (65.5%) in the 'ambient group', compared with 4 (13.3%) in the standard group, reported spending less than half of their time in the standard labour bed. (This does imply that women did not spend all their labour in the ambient room.) Twelve women allocated to the ambient room had artificial oxytocin infusions, compared with 21 allocated to the standard room. She considered this a good basis to go on to do an RCT.

The problems with trials

Childbirth is not a condition that lends itself well to randomised controlled trials. It is easy to see that administering a drug is a treatment, an active intervention, but it is difficult to manipulate other aspects of birth such as position in labour and birth in such a way that one can be sure that the aspect under investigation is the only variable. Position in labour concerns human behaviour, the behaviour of the woman – does she want to be told what position to adopt? – and the behaviour of the caregiver – will the caregiver cooperate with the researcher in encouraging or discouraging a particular position? Research into position in childbirth was possible only because women's behaviour was already highly controlled in the hospital setting. Position could be studied by asking caregivers to encourage or discourage certain behaviours, by relaxing constraints on movement, by providing alternative furniture and by changing the means by which the fetus was monitored. When position for labour and birth was subjected to clinical trials, the upright position was deemed the experimental condition, care on the bed as standard.

Position in labour should not be under the control of the caregiver but of the woman herself. A woman may be randomised to the 'upright' arm of a trial but may not 'comply'; she may choose to lie down. Some trials state the amount of time actually spent upright or walking and it is usually a small percentage of the total time in labour. Results are analysed under 'intention to treat' and all results are analysed, including those of women who do not comply. One of the earlier trials of position in labour (Díaz et al, 1980) cannot be used as evidence for a Cochrane review because the women who did not comply were taken out of the study group. The motivation for the Díaz study seems to have been to change the hospital practice of confining all women to bed for labour in order to encourage more 'native' women to choose hospital birth: '…native women often reject the lying-down position when it is imposed. This has given rise to unnecessary problems in the acceptance of medical care by certain native people' (the study was done in South America). The researchers analysed only the data from women in the experimental group who had remained sitting, standing or walking for the whole first stage (from 4-5 cm to 10 cm dilatation). Removing the 79 women who must have taken to the bed at some stage invalidated the results which otherwise showed an impressive reduction in the length of the first stage of labour and a reduction in forceps delivery. Another very interesting paper that falls outside the parameters for a Cochrane review because it is not an RCT is by Méndez-Bauer et al (1975). This will be considered in more detail later on in this book. Ideally, the variables to be compared in an RCT should not be horizontal or vertical positions, but rather choice of position versus no choice of position.

It may be as unhelpful to prevent a woman from lying down if she wants to as it may be to prevent her from being upright. Moreover, choice of position may be meaningless if the furniture in the room favours one position over another.

Despite all the limitations of the currently available literature, the RCTs published to date have shown that in hospital labour and birth is usually shorter and less painful when women use upright positions. This information is repeated again and again throughout the literature, whether written for women, for midwives or even for the medical profession. The clinical evidence on upright positions in the first stage of labour is full and unequivocal. It is already disseminated as best practice by institutions such as the World Health Organisation (WHO), the Royal College of Obstetricians and Gynaecologists (RCOG) and the Royal College of Midwives (RCM).

The RCOG's recommended advice in 2009 agrees with Cochrane:

The Royal College of Obstetricians and Gynaecologists (RCOG) encourages women to mobilise and remain upright as much as possible during the first stage of labour. It is likely that being upright helps that [sic] baby's head to descend and turn into the right position. The pressure of the baby's head on the cervix may also help to strengthen contractions…

All women having a vaginal birth are encouraged to ambulate during the first stage of labour, provided that they feel capable of doing so. The RCOG recommends that women be encouraged to assume whatever position is most comfortable to them.

It is encouraging that the RCOG recognises the benefit of labouring upright for all women having a vaginal birth even though the Cochrane review had looked mainly at low-risk women. This endorsement from the RCOG means that effectively there are virtually no contra-indications to upright position in the first stage of labour, so it is hard to understand why the bed still takes pride of place in the labour rooms on obstetric units.

The World Health Organisation (Makuch, 2010) is also notionally in favour of the upright position but its statement does not go so far as the RCOG:

The duration of the first stage of labour may be reduced by about one hour in women who maintain the upright position and walk around; they are also likely to receive less epidural analgesia. Since the review did not find any adverse effects associated with remaining upright, health-care professionals and facilities *may encourage* [my italics] labouring women to adopt positions that women are most comfortable with.

The WHO bases its guidance largely on obstetric opinion and there is evidence of obstetric bias in its statement in the very weak advice to encourage upright position (*may encourage*). The reason for this may lie in the powerful obstetric lobby influencing the WHO. Compared to obstetricians in the USA, British obstetricians are positively enlightened. In the USA, obstetricians, anaesthetists, hospitals and drug companies would lose income if more women were able to adopt comfortable positions in labour. If any other benign obstetric intervention had been shown to reduce the length of the first stage and reduce the need for epidural anaesthesia without having any adverse effects, it would have been worded more strongly. The WHO is happy to leave control over women's position to the convenience of the healthcare professionals. It concerns me greatly that the western world is still exporting bed-based obstetrics to countries with high maternal mortality rates.

RCM Better Births Initiative

Instead of just issuing a position statement, the Royal College of Midwives has attempted to change practice. In its *Guidelines on Positions for Labour and Birth*, it says that midwives should be proactive in demonstrating and encouraging different positions. It recognises the main barriers: firstly, that women choose to do what is expected of them and they expect to labour on the bed; secondly, that the environment may lack suitable furniture; and thirdly, that other interventions such as intravenous drips, fetal monitors and epidural anaesthesia adversely affect women's mobility. Midwives have the best opportunity to encourage women to change their position in labour because they spend the most time caring for women in labour, but many midwives have themselves been influenced by the prevailing hospital culture that sees women as patients. Midwives come under strong peer pressure to conform to usual hospital practice. Those encouraging active birth may be ridiculed by their colleagues (Russell, 2011).

UK national guidelines (NICE)

The National Institute on Health and Care Excellence (NICE) has a guideline on the care of healthy women and their babies during childbirth (Clinical Guideline 55) but a guideline for women expected to have problems will not be available until 2015; it must be presumed that for the moment the guideline includes all women not having a planned caesarean section. Under the first section, communication, caregivers are asked to 'encourage the woman to adapt the environment to meet her individual needs' and in the second section, throughout labour, the guideline asks caregivers to 'encourage the woman to mobilise and adopt comfortable positions'. The first mention of the upright position itself is for the second stage when it advises: 'Discourage the woman from lying supine/semi-supine. Consider the woman's position, hydration and pain-relief needs'. It also mentions upright position in its advice on epidurals: 'Encourage and help the woman to adopt any comfortable upright position. Consider the woman's position, hydration and pain-relief needs.' However, it fails to mention upright position in its advice on delay in the first or the second stage of labour, despite research evidence showing that the upright position shortens both first and second stage of labour.

What actually happens

Given the strength of the clinical evidence favouring upright position for labour and birth this evidence is remarkably low key and the failure to give stronger advice is reflected in the results of a survey conducted by the Care Quality Commission in 2013. It found that only 71% of women were able to move around and choose the position that made them most comfortable most of the time, with 21% saying they could do this some of the time and 8% saying they were never able to do this. Eighty-five per cent gave birth on a bed, and 8% gave birth in water. Five per cent of women gave birth on their side, 26% were lying or lying supported by pillows, and 32% had their legs in stirrups. There was an increase in the proportion of women giving birth on their backs in stirrups compared with three years previously but there was also an increase in the number of women giving birth while kneeling, squatting or standing (16%).

In the USA the picture is less bright. A survey of 2,400 mothers found that only two out of five women walked around once they were admitted to the hospital and regular contractions had begun. More than two-thirds (68%) of women who gave birth vaginally reported that they lay on their backs while giving birth, while 23% indicated they gave birth in a propped up (semi-sitting) position. Three per cent gave birth on their side while only 5% gave birth on hands and knees or in an upright position (Transforming Maternity Care, 2013).

Conclusion

There is abundant evidence that an upright position in the first stage of labour is beneficial to the mother. She is more comfortable, has less pain, and labour is shorter. For the second stage of labour there may be some drawbacks. Average blood loss is greater only by 60 ml, although midwives think this is because it is easier to measure and women are more likely to have a second-degree tear although less likely to have an episiotomy. Women are less uncomfortable, can tolerate pain better and have less difficulty in pushing the baby out. Women in the upright groups also expressed a preference for the upright posture for their next birth. There is a lower rate of forceps delivery.

Perhaps it is equally important that women should feel in control of the birth of their baby. In a paper on alternative birth positions written for *Canadian Family Physician* in 1988, Reid and Harris write that 'because the upright woman can see and be seen, she is more likely to be spoken to and be actively involved in the process ... attendants are encouraged to treat her as a person, since she is not in a passive or subordinate posture.' They point out that all upright positions are less convenient for the operator, especially if he or she is attempting an instrumental delivery. Perhaps the proportion of women giving birth in 'alternative' positions in hospital reflects the quality of evidence-based maternity care in that hospital. I look forward to the day when the supine position is consigned to the history books.

4 The active uterus

In order to understand why the mother's position is so important in labour it is useful to know how the uterus works and what stops it working, what makes contractions painful and what makes them bearable. I want to get you to see the uterus in a new more powerful light, as an organ that women are blessed with which works dynamically to birth her baby in the best possible way for both.

The uterus is the most amazing part of the human body; we underestimate it. It has evolved to have two diametrically opposite functions, the first to be a safe haven for the fetus for the nine months of pregnancy – incubation – and the second to propel the baby into the outside world – ejection. During labour it has to fulfil both functions at one and the same time, truly miraculous. And what's more it can repeat the process again and again over the woman's reproductive lifetime of 30 years or so. In this chapter I hope to get you to see the uterus with different eyes, as an organ exquisitely designed by evolution to nurture and then give birth to the next generation. I want women to be proud of the life-giving organ within them instead of blaming it for every manner of ill from hysteria to caesarean section. If the uterus fails to do its work properly it is usually because we have stopped it working as it evolved to work, we have interfered with its function by forcing it into labour too soon, by not giving it the freedom of movement it requires to work or by disrupting the finely balanced hormones of labour that regulate its work. A better understanding of how the uterus works should lead to better care.

It says so much about the miraculous nature of the uterus that the three objects I choose for illustration are so far removed from each other that it is impossible to picture a conglomerate of them.

In form the uterus has much in common with the party balloon; in function it is both an incubator and an ejection seat – although the uterus is unique in managing to propel the fragile baby outside the body while itself remaining inside the body. I've used the word 'propel' deliberately – it gives the impression of a quick process and I believe that the body has to work hard to slow down this automatic ejection reflex process to make labour safe for mother and baby once labour has eventually kicked off. This may seem counterintuitive – we are more used to thinking that human labour is a long slow painful process – but I believe that the hormonal forces that evolved to allow a habitually upright walking mammal to remain pregnant against the forces of gravity had to be stronger than the hormonal forces required for those mammals which spend most of their time on all fours.

Not only does the uterus fulfil the function of both incubator and ejector seat in labour, but it can repeat the whole process twenty or more times in a woman's lifetime. Modern technology has given us the incubator and ejection seat within the last 100 years but evolution has been working on the mammalian uterus for 200 million years, the primate uterus for about 70 million years and the human uterus for about one million years (Pilbeam, 1972) and, if we allow it to, it usually works beautifully.

The uterus is the most powerful and underestimated organ in the body; before pregnancy it weighs 60 g, by the time of birth it weighs 1 kg and it reverts to its pre-pregnancy weight by six weeks after the birth. It is by far the strongest muscle in the body, exerting a pressure of up to 120mmHg

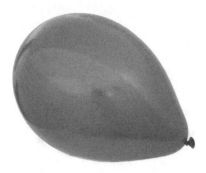

Figure 15: The uterus is a balloon.

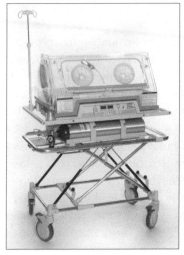

Figure 16: The uterus is an incubator.

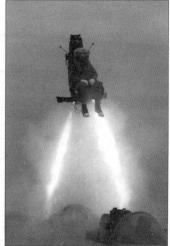

Figure 17: The uterus is an ejection seat.

during the first stage of labour, to which can be added another 30mmHg of pressure during second stage as the woman uses her abdominal muscles to exert even more pressure.

Evolution of the uterus

150 million years ago or more the uterus evolved from the oviducts which expelled eggs into the outside world. The uterus was formed at the junction of the tubes from the two ovaries; it evolved to delay the egg on its journey to the outside world and to incubate the fertilised egg within the body. At around the same time in evolutionary history, natural selection found a new use for a biochemical which had previously been merely one step of a metabolic pathway in the biosynthesis of the steroid hormones, cortisol, oestrogen and testosterone, from the common precursor molecule, cholesterol. That 'new' hormone was progesterone and was named for its best known function – pro (for) gestation (pregnancy). Its mode of action is to prepare the uterus to receive an egg and to communicate the possibility of pregnancy to the brain and switch the whole female body to pregnancy mode.

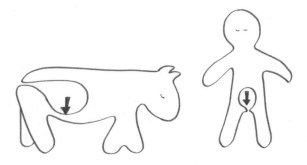

Figure 18: The hormonal mechanical forces of the human female body have to work hard at maintaining pregnancy (incubation) against the forces of gravity which would lead to premature birth (ejection). All that is required for labour to start is for the forces of pregnancy to be relaxed to allow nature to take its course.

Form

- *The muscle of the uterus is a hollow elastic bag.* The uterus is made of smooth muscle, the type of muscle which forms tubes and bags in the body, such as blood vessels, the bladder, intestines and bowel. The life processes performed by these organs 'run' in the background all the time, smooth muscle contracts constantly and requires no conscious input to do its work. What is different about the uterus (and other reproductive smooth muscle such as the male vas deferens) is that contractions can occasionally become strong enough to be felt – at orgasm, at menstruation and in giving birth.

  Smooth muscle isn't under voluntary control, it is under control of the autonomic nervous system and is sensitive to many different hormones. Generally speaking progesterone and stress hormones such as adrenaline tend to stop the uterus contracting, while oestrogen, oxytocin and prostaglandins tend to promote contractions (Buckley, 2002). Stress hormones tend to down-regulate oxytocin. Keeping a woman free of stress in labour is a good way to improve uterine function and reduce pain.

  Another way to improve function and reduce pain is to find

good positions for labour. The uterus has to 'know' where to contract in order to steer the fetus to the outlet. Unlike a party balloon, the uterus is not an inert, passive elastic bag floating aimlessly about in space but it both contains the body of the fetus and is contained inside the mother's body and has to fit around other organs in her pelvis and abdomen. Most importantly as far as maternal position is concerned, its physical relationship to the mother's spine must be taken into account; strong though the uterus is, it is unable to push through bone! The uterus responds dynamically to maternal and fetal physical and emotional stimulation: it uses physical, hormonal and nervous signals from the mother, and physical and hormonal signals from the fetus.

Of all the signals to contract, the response of the uterus to being stretched is probably the most important as far as position in labour is concerned. After all, the process of birth is the physical movement of a physical body in a particular direction out of another physical body. The uterus has to 'know' where to contract to steer the fetus in the right direction.

- *It's about the same size as a balloon when a woman is not pregnant* The uterus can generate more of itself; it grows from 60 g to 1 kg during pregnancy and then within six weeks of birth it digests itself to go back nearly to its pre-pregnancy state. To grow a baby the uterus needs to grow. Throughout pregnancy the uterus stretches to accommodate the growing fetus. The uterus is an elastic bag that expands as the fetus grows. Paradoxically, part of that growth could be owed to the very stretching itself; stretching uterine muscle leads to contraction (Wray, 1993) and any muscle that is 'worked' becomes stronger and increases in size – the uterus is unlikely to be an exception to this rule. During pregnancy the muscle contractions that are happening all the time to individual muscle cells do not lead to labour because the hormone progesterone stops them joining forces and working together thus preventing the uterus contracting as a whole. The hormones of pregnancy also encourage growth. Individual muscle cells grow to ten times their original size. The number of muscle cells also increases.

- *It's flat with touching sides when empty and pear-shaped when 'full'.*
- *After being stretched, it will revert to its original shape – it has elastic memory.* Imagine putting your fist against a blown-up balloon, then withdrawing it – the balloon regains its pear shape. You can do this to a balloon from the outside but the fetus will do it from the inside. The uterus is more dynamic than a balloon; during labour the muscle cells of the uterus react to being stretched by becoming even smaller – contraction leads to retraction.
- *It can expand to many times its original size and then revert to near its previous size.* Deflated balloons never quite retain their virgin state; neither does the uterus.
- *It can be under enormous pressure and yet not burst.*
- *Up to a certain point it can cope with slight flaws in its substance.* The uterus can, for example, cope with scar tissue from a caesarean section – but you can never quite tell.
- *It is fragile yet immensely strong.*
- *If maltreated it can burst.*
- *It can be tied shut.* Obstetricians can quite literally tie the uterus shut with a Sirodhka stitch to retain its contents.
- *Undo the knot and it will deflate.*

The cervix – the neck of the balloon

If the main body of the uterus is like a balloon and is an incubator, then the cervix is the escape hatch and the knot. It is about three centimetres long. The top of the cervical canal is within the uterus, the lower end protrudes into the top of the vagina. The uterus is rather more elaborate than a party balloon which is made of a single piece of latex. While all the muscle of the uterus is the same, it is thicker in some places than others. It is thickest at the top, the fundus, and thinnest at the bottom, the cervix.

The cervix needs reinforcement to ensure that it stays shut; only 10–15% of the substance of the cervix is muscle. The main component is rigid collagen embedded in a biological gel-like substance (Bauer *et al*, 2007). The collagen fibres are aligned longitudinally on the inside of the cervix while the muscle at the cervix goes round the circumference. It is only when the collagen column at the cervix is broken down and the cervix softens that the cervical muscle can be stretched and the door can start to open to unleash the full power of the labouring uterus.

The uterus itself has to stretch during pregnancy to accommodate the growing fetus but the cervix is stretch resistant. With the unyielding collagen matrix in position, the cervix cannot stretch enough for labour to start. Even when there is a discernible opening, as there often is towards the end of pregnancy, and even during early labour, the uterus will not 'empty itself' so long as the rigid collagen is still in place. As a last precaution against precipitate labour, cervical muscle can contract to keep itself closed – it can contract even in the early stages of spontaneous labour, although it is more likely to contract to try and maintain pregnancy during an induced labour (Olah, Gee and Brown, 1993).

The incubator

The incubator is the man-made item that needs the least explanation as it is designed to do a small part of the same work as the woman-made version, although it will never come any way near to matching what a mother's body and her baby's placenta co-operate to do automatically. Huxley's *Brave New World* with its rooms full of incubating babies is still a figment of the imagination and women who wish to bypass pregnancy and have a baby that bears their genes have to undergo the enforced superovulation of IVF to give up their eggs and borrow another woman's body for a surrogate pregnancy.

The lifeline
The uterus provides a safe, warm, enclosed environment to grow a baby. The baby supplies his own line-in and line-out

– the umbilical cord, which is attached to the placenta, and serves as the interface between mother and baby. Oxygen and nutrients from the mother are transferred by simple diffusion across the placenta and the placenta also provides a route for the fetus to get rid of waste products.

The placenta is also an endocrine gland, a means of hormonal communication between mother and fetus. During pregnancy it takes over many hormone-regulating functions from the mother's hypothalamus, chiefly the secretion of gonadotropin-releasing hormone (GnRH) which controls oestrogen secretion, but also other regulating hormones such as thyrotropin-releasing hormone (TRH) which regulates thyroid hormones. The placenta is dictatorial, for example the placenta secretes the human chorionic gonadotropin (hCG), the hormone which instructs the ovary to continue to produce progesterone, the pro-pregnancy hormone, and to stop its monthly cycle. Human placental lactogen (HPL) tells the mother to prepare her breasts for lactation. The placenta instructs the mother to increase her blood sugar levels to supply the fetus with glucose, and it passes back waste products for the mother to excrete. The placenta 'orders' what the fetus needs the mother's blood to supply. It scoops up her antibodies and passes them on to her baby, giving passive immunity to the baby to see him through the first few months of life and it acts as a barrier to many blood-borne microbes (although some infectious diseases such as rubella and HIV can still be passed on). The placenta hides the genetic identity of the fetus from the mother's immune system so she does not reject her fetus as a foreign body. The placenta also provides a reservoir of the fetus' own blood.

I can't resist putting in a picture (overleaf) of an infant attached to his placenta. Of course the placenta isn't really a parachute but, together with the umbilical cord, it does function as the fetal lifeline all the way through pregnancy, labour and a few minutes after birth while the newborn baby is still receiving his own blood from his placenta. The various inputs that Sarah, the cartoonist, has shown could be thought of as holes in the parachute silk. Each unnecessary intervention in labour can compromise the fetal lifeline and can make landing that much more tricky.

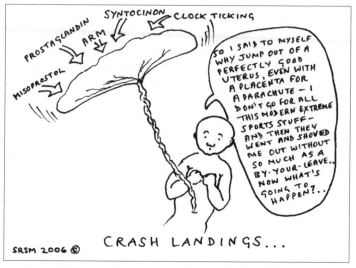

Figure 19: The site where the placenta is attached could be anywhere but is usually at the level of the middle of the uterus; too high up and it tends to make contractions less efficient, too low down and it risks blocking the exit or separating too soon which leads to maternal haemorrhage.

Ejection seat

The ejection seat is the most masculine of the three images I have chosen to explain the function of the uterus. The man-made ejection seat is designed to come right out of an aircraft which might crash at any minute. Its purpose is simple – to eject the pilot straight out of the aircraft to a safe distance. The pilot then deploys a parachute to allow him to land safely on the ground. I've left this metaphor until last because it is a frightening image; ejection seats are activated only when something catastrophic has gone wrong with the aircraft. The metaphor holds for the uterus when labour is premature; premature labour can be triggered through fetal distress or maternal distress or both. Fetal stress hormones also have a role to play in normal labour at term (Liggins, 1969).

I needed a very powerful metaphor for the work of the uterus in giving birth, if only to counteract the images I have used above, the 'fluffy' party balloon and the incubator which allows a helpless infant to cling on to life in the absence of his mother. The uterus is the most powerful muscle in the human body and is designed by natural selection to push a baby out into the world. A man-made ejection seat can be used only once and, along with its passenger, it is ejected clear of the aircraft, but it pales into insignificance beside the female uterus which fashions itself around the needs of the fetus, pushes it out while remaining inside the mother's body, and then shrinks down again within six weeks of birth only to go through the whole process again for the next baby.

The seat itself

Pilots are already sitting in the seat that will eject them if they need to bail out, but the fetus has to get himself into the best position for leaving his mother's body. Towards the end of pregnancy and in early labour the baby must be manoeuvred into the optimal position for birth. This is one of the most important but least appreciated aspects of labour. Human childbirth is more painful and difficult than birth in other primate species because, unlike other species of ape, there is not a straightforward exit from the mother's body. Much of the work of labour involves getting the baby into the best possible position to leave his mother's body. If this aspect of labour was better understood, labour rooms everywhere would have all sorts of furniture to support labouring women and most would get rid of the bed altogether.

Escape hatch

Before an ejection seat can operate, an escape hatch in the fuselage of the aircraft must be opened. The other part of the work of the uterus in the first stage of labour is to open the escape hatch of the cervix. In an aircraft the pilot has a button to press which will open the escape hatch quickly. However, the female body takes far longer to open the escape hatch than it does to 'eject' the baby. The first stage of labour takes hours if not days, the second stage usually takes around an hour, while the third stage (expelling the placenta) takes minutes.

How does the uterus work?

The background contractions that have been occurring throughout pregnancy are not strong enough to attract a woman's attention but at some stage in pregnancy many women become aware of Braxton Hicks contractions, in which the uterus becomes hard for a few seconds then relaxes again. Such contractions can be triggered by a full bladder or a change in the position of the fetus. If a section of uterus is stretched – from the outside by a full bladder or from the inside by a moving fetus – all the stretched muscle cells will tend to contract together. In a tubular structure such as the gut or blood vessels the effect is to move substances along the tube, like squeezing a tube of toothpaste, but in the closed system of the uterus, during pregnancy, contractions will be strong enough to fold the baby back into the fetal position after he has stretched himself. Local stretch will lead to local contraction but the contraction will not spread beyond the stretched tissue. In order to contract as a coordinated whole, muscle contractions need to be synchronised. Contractions need to be able to spread throughout the whole uterus and work together.

During the last three to four weeks of pregnancy the cervix prepares to open. The process is termed 'ripening' and involves dissolving the collagen scaffolding of the cervix which softens it. Naturally secreted prostaglandins break down collagen and lead to cervical ripening. (Prostaglandin gels can be administered to induce labour.) Thus the first indication that labour might be imminent may be a change in vaginal secretions. The collagen matrix in which the cervical muscle is embedded breaks down, partially untying the hormonal knot. This process can go on over a number of days. The breakdown of collagen results in a watery discharge, known to some midwives as a 'cervical weep', which can perhaps be confused with the waters breaking (Evans, 2012). As the cervix becomes less rigid a 'plug' of mucus may loosen and be discharged – termed a 'show'.

Soon afterwards the uterus will be making its presence known to its owner. Contractions which have been taking place throughout pregnancy will now become strong enough to be felt and strong enough to start pulling up the cervix which will transform the uterus from a balloon to a tunnel. If the baby or the cervix are not already lined up well with the rest of the tunnel to the outside world, these contractions must also align the baby and the cervix with the exit.

Thinking about it using just plain physics, and thinking about the uterus as a closed system, as it is during pregnancy, even if contractions could spread far and wide, all that they would achieve is to contract to make a smaller pear-shaped container. Actually, Braxton Hicks contractions do start to spread and this is what happens. Towards the end of pregnancy there are four things that happen to change the situation and tip a woman's body into labour and I'm not sure that we know, or indeed if it makes much difference, which of the four events comes first:

1. First the knot is untied, the cervix ripens and becomes softer, losing its scaffolding of collagen. Now the uterus is no longer a closed system; the cervix is the point of least resistance and any contractions higher up than the cervix itself will try to force it to open. However, there is still some resistance; the muscle at the cervix is circular muscle, if it contracts it will still try to keep the exit route closed. The sides of the neck of the womb are still close together, if not actually touching. If the fetus has adopted the 'textbook' position, he is lying head down just above the top of the cervix, the internal os, about three centimetres above his exit from the uterus. We will leave him here for a bit, poised to begin his journey into the outside world.

The other three things that happen both concern the biochemical environment of the uterus.

2. Oestrogen levels rise towards the end of pregnancy and oestrogen 'wires up' the uterus for labour. Oestrogen promotes the secretion of a protein called connexin-43 which could be thought of as 'living wire' linking uterine cells together into a network and enabling the uterus to contract as a whole. Now a contraction can spread

from a stretched area to an unstretched area (Lefebvre, 1995). The electrical activity of muscle cell contracting in one place will spread outwards, travelling along the connexin 'wires'. The contracting area can now communicate with other muscle cells.

3. Oxytocin is a protein hormone secreted by the pituitary gland and has been known to cause contractions of the uterus since 1906. It was first synthesised in 1953 and has long been used in obstetrics to speed up labour. Artificial oxytocin is known as Syntocinon in the UK and Pitocin in the USA. Hormones are chemical messengers. In order for oxytocin to have any biological effect at a particular site in the body that site must contain oxytocin receptors. (You could think of the pituitary gland as a radio transmitter, transmitting the oxytocin signal, and the oxytocin receptors as being radio receivers, the greater the number of radios, the louder the noise.) Oestrogen increases the number of oxytocin receptors at the uterus. This means that the same dose of oxytocin will have more places to act and will therefore have a stronger effect. (Oxytocin blood levels do not change during the first stage of labour. The available oxytocin simply has more places in which it can act. Normal labour does not require high doses of oxytocin.)

4. Calcium is the 'fuel' that makes the uterine muscle cells contract but the 'fuel tank' is outside the cell itself. There is more calcium in the spaces *between* cells than there is *inside* the cell. Oestrogen increases the number of calcium channels in the uterine muscle cell membranes allowing more 'fuel' into the cell. A greater number of calcium channels means that cells can refuel more quickly. Individual uterine muscle cells are thus able to contract more frequently.

The net result of all these hormonal changes is that the biomechanical properties of the uterine muscle tissue change. The uterus will react more strongly to oxytocin because there are more oxytocin receptors to pick up the signal. Contractions will spread further because muscle cells have become linked into an electrical network and, having more available fuel, cells will 'fire' at a faster rate. The uterus starts to act as an open system instead of a closed system. Now when part of the uterus is stretched, contractions will spread outward beyond the stretched portion. If the baby is not yet in the best position to start his journey, these stronger contractions can help position him (which can be a long and painful process if the mother cannot move). The uterus will start to open at the point of least resistance, the cervix. Once the baby has fitted his head into this mother's pelvis he is poised to begin his journey through the pelvis.

I believe that the uterus will work much more efficiently and effectively if it is ready to labour. While it is possible to force a uterus into labour using artificial hormones, it is much better to wait until it has been primed for labour and can work as a coordinated whole as nature intended.

5 The choreography of the uterus in labour and birth

I have really struggled over the years to uncover how the uterus works as a whole and I'm still learning. There is still very little information in the childbirth literature; most sources merely describe *what* happens: i.e. contractions are felt, they get stronger and closer together until the cervix effaces (thins out) and opens. This is the first stage of labour. Then there may be a 'rest and be thankful' phase after which contractions start again. During the second stage of labour, the mother adds voluntary abdominal effort to each contraction and pushes her baby out. Then comes the third stage of labour where contractions start again and the placenta is delivered. Obstetric textbooks talk about the three Ps: the Powers – the force of uterine contractions; the Passage – the birth canal; and the Passenger – the fetus. The mother herself, although the owner of the uterus providing the power, does not appear in the obstetric account of labour. A midwifery website puts her back into the picture (www.coursewareobjects, Lowdermilk, accessed 2014) by adding two more Ps: Position of the mother and Psychological responses of the mother. Perhaps we should add the Placenta which provides the fetal lifeline throughout labour. In this chapter I am trying to tie all these Ps together to produce a clearer picture of the physiology of labour. (I object to describing the baby as a passenger when he actively participates in his own birth, and I'm uncomfortable with calling him a fetus. I think I'll start calling him the baby in this chapter.)

I must start with a warning, as much to myself as my readers. Armstrong and Feldman (2007) say that:

> ...childbirth is infinitely dynamic. We cannot adequately understand it by naming anatomical parts and describing

physiological processes, nor are we done when we describe its choreography. Birth functions in the context of mind and spirit. They act directly on birth and give it the complexity we associate with life.

I am aware that, in looking at the choreography of labour and trying to analyse the biomechanics of the uterus, I am groping towards an understanding of labour which has eluded generations of childbirth educators. I believe that by looking after the mother's mind and spirit, you *are* looking after her body and her baby – until her baby is born there is no other way that you can look after him. So while this chapter is focused on one part of her body, her uterus, it goes without saying that it is set in the context of the rest of her body and her mind and her spirit.

If you are a healthcare professional, you may not agree with a lay person taking on such a task but it's worth a try and is unlikely to do any harm. At least my mind isn't cluttered up with what I'm supposed to think and I have the advantage of knowing what it *feels like* to labour. I now know that my first labour would have been terrible had I not been allowed to move as I wanted. If nothing else, this chapter will get you thinking.

Labour is a *pas de deux* between the mother and the baby: during the first stage of labour the uterus is the interface between their two bodies; during second stage her vagina is the interface and at last she can feel her baby directly. The mother can move, the baby can move. Contractions don't 'just happen'; the uterus contracts when it receives signals to contract. Knowing the anatomical and physiological underpinnings of the dance of labour may be crucial when considering what women need in order to have a good labour. I originally wrote that the beauty of physiology is that it doesn't go out of date very much, we just learn more about it and build on previous knowledge, but I'm coming to the conclusion that we have got some of it so very wrong that we have been haring off down the wrong road for the last 60 years. That road has led to a situation where in the UK only 60% of women report having a normal birth, with 25% giving birth by caesarean section and 15% having an instrumental delivery. I think the blame can be laid at the feet of clinicians who have a very poor understanding of normal physiology and no idea of the physical and emotional needs of women in labour.

The work of a woman's body in the first stage of labour is involuntary, automatic. In one sense, contractions do 'just happen' in that they cannot be made to occur through an act of will on the part of the mother. However, just because a woman cannot 'will' a contraction to happen, we must get ourselves out of the rather defeatist way of thinking that there is nothing she can do voluntarily to change the strength, effectiveness or the pain of her contractions. Whether a woman has an easy labour or a hard labour is not just a matter of luck. Excruciating pain is not inevitable and drugs are not the only answer to pain. Relaxation and breathing techniques don't just allow the labouring mother to cope with what clinicians see as inescapable pain, they help to alter the way the uterus is working to make contractions less painful. Some pain is avoidable. A uterus that is working efficiently – as it was 'designed' to work – will produce contraction patterns that steer the baby to the outside world. Women's birth stories show again and again that, on the whole, effective coordinated contractions are less painful than ineffective uncoordinated contractions. The rule of thumb for mothers to experience efficient, bearable contractions is to try to find a position that relieves pain. The contracting uterus is housed within a body and a mother can move her body. The standard hospital response to pain is to offer pain-relieving drugs or epidural anaesthesia to block the pain. When under the influence of drugs, the mother may be too doped up to act on positional signals; when the pain is blocked she cannot even feel them.

Position matters

Méndez-Bauer, a doctor, became interested in maternal position in labour when his wife gave birth. The hospital where she gave birth required her to lie down and, as a medic himself, he was unable to explain to her why his colleagues insisted on the supine position. He became fascinated with the subject. In 1975 with the help of colleagues he studied contraction patterns in 20 first-time mothers who had gone into labour spontaneously with the baby in the vertex (head first) position. The women were asked to alternate their position between standing and supine at 30-minute intervals. Intrauterine pressure monitoring recordings showed that contractions were more intense in the standing position; 19 out of 20 women found them less painful. (The contractions were measured in the most accurate way by a pressure catheter placed inside the uterus.)

Stronger contractions are thus *not* necessarily more painful. The authors also found significant changes in the frequency of contractions for seven women. 'In six of them, the frequency of contractions diminished when the patient changed from supine to standing position and it increased in the remaining one'. This challenges the classic view that contractions get progressively stronger and closer together during labour. Although women had fewer contractions, the contractions were more effective.

The authors asked the women about both comfort and pain. All women except one found standing more comfortable and all (except the woman who said there was no difference in comfort) reported less pain or no difference when standing. Average duration of labour between 3 and 10 cm dilatation was just under four hours (3 h 55 mins +/-1 h 40 mins) which is very much shorter than that reported in an obstetric textbook of the time (6 hours 20 mins; Cibils, 1972). In the standing position women had fewer, less painful, more comfortable contractions which achieved as good as or better total uterine pressure over time (see Figures 21 and 22, page 85). The paper restricts itself to two positions and says nothing about the stances adopted by the standing women, or the furniture used to help them maintain a standing position, but we must assume that they had some way of supporting themselves.

In the discussion section of the paper the authors highlight three statements: 'the periods of standing position could be a factor contributing to the shorter duration of labour; the standing position did not have any undesirable effect on the fetus or newborn; and there appear to be no clear arguments against the use of standing position during labour.'

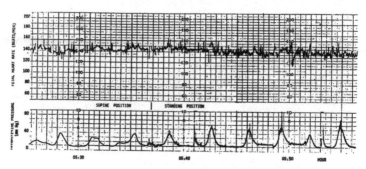

Figure 20: Cardiotocogram of fetal heart rate (FHR) and contraction pattern of a first-time mother labouring in two different positions. The recording shows the patterns before and after a change of position when the mother was half way to full dilatation. 'Note the increase in the intensity of contractions in standing position as well as less irregularities, suggesting a better coordination.' (Méndez-Bauer, 1975)

Although no expert in cardiotocography (CTG) interpretation I find these print outs (Figure 20) compelling and wonder how the caregivers could have continued with the study when the supine position showed such a clear disadvantage on the CTG recordings or, indeed, why the women agreed to change back to the supine position after 30 minutes of labouring upright. (But they were patients in a hospital and patients tend to do what they are told!) This was not a randomised controlled trial (RCT); each woman acted as her own control. However, the evidence from RCTs summarised in Chapter Three also shows that maternal position in the first and second stages of labour affects progress; labour is shorter and there is less need for pain relief and operative delivery.

Pain signals

The most obvious way the brain has to influence a mother's position is to use pain signals. Just as it is in any other situation, the biological purpose of pain in labour must be to elicit pain-avoiding behaviour. Before analgesics and anaesthesia were available, the resources of the body itself had to be mobilised to relieve or avoid pain – much of the advice from midwives and the natural childbirth movement for reducing or coping with pain is based on the body and the mind: find a comfortable

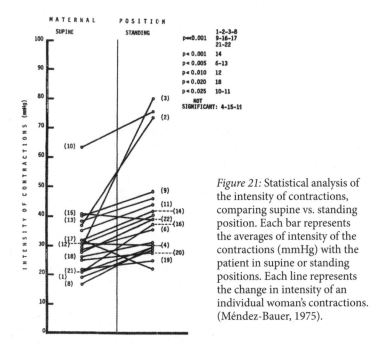

Figure 21: Statistical analysis of the intensity of contractions, comparing supine vs. standing position. Each bar represents the averages of intensity of the contractions (mmHg) with the patient in supine or standing positions. Each line represents the change in intensity of an individual woman's contractions. (Méndez-Bauer, 1975).

Figure 22: Statistical analysis of the frequency of contractions, comparing supine vs. standing position. The frequency is measured as the number of contractions present in 10 minutes. Each bar shows the change in frequency for one woman. (Méndez-Bauer, 1975)

position, try using the birth pool, relax, rub here, press there, breathe through, 'don't panic'. All these techniques use the body's own resources to alleviate pain.

Instinct

The primary instinct in birth must surely be activity to avoid or relieve pain. If women are unable to act on their instincts, birth will be more painful than it needs to be; this is the case when labour takes place on the bed, which greatly limits a woman's options for instinctive movement. The attitude from many health professionals, and the world at large, is that agonising pain during childbirth is inevitable. Such an attitude leads to the assumption that it is inhuman to deny pain relief, but many women prefer not to take drugs in labour if they can avoid them. Finding comfortable positions helps to alleviate pain or, at the very least, enables women to cope with it. Pain can be reduced by concentrating on where contractions are happening, by 'listening to' the body's instructions, by relaxation, by careful breathing. The diaphragm is just above the uterus. Slow regular breathing may interfere least with uterine function; panicky breathing in gulps will add another layer of physical interference.

Instinctive movement during labour may also happen below the threshold of consciousness. In everyday life people change their posture all the time to maintain comfortable positions, and we rarely sit completely still. Why should the body behave any differently in labour? Usually we are completely unaware of these small movements. We don't have to get as far as feeling pain before responding automatically to signals to move. The proof of this is the one time when it doesn't work, when we get pins and needles because the blood supply and nerves – and pain signals – have been temporarily blocked; the pain is worse as sensation is returning. The above relates to skeletal movements but there is no reason why internal organs should not also elicit bodily movement. Consider that one usually has time enough to get to a suitable place before vomiting – the 'about to be sick' feeling (as opposed to vague feelings of nausea) precedes the dash to the loo. Apologies for grossness, but next time your bowel works try to take notice of the way you move about on the toilet seat to allow efficient expulsion!

Usually the movement required is fairly small but in labour it could be quite large. Jane Evans, a midwife skilled in the care of women with breech babies (who are coming bottom first), has closely observed many women as they give birth and has noticed that there are certain movements women make automatically as the baby is moving through the pelvis if they are on all fours, a position that gives them freedom of movement (Evans, 2012). She attributes these movements to parts of the baby impinging on maternal nerves. If breech birth elicits a specific set of movements, it is likely that similar movements will happen during births where the baby is coming head first. I am talking of subtle movements here, but occasionally large movements may be required and the subconscious brain seems to be able to communicate directly in something like words. This happened to me just before the birth of my third baby. I was conscious of an overwhelming instruction from my own brain to get up out of my forward kneeling position on the floor and move onto the bed. This was directly opposed to my plans for the birth – I had made sure that the midwife brought her birthing stool ready for the birth itself. Almost as soon as I had laid down on my right side on the bed, I started to push my baby out. I'm wondering now whether it was this profound 'right brain' experience that gave me such a passion to explore the physiology and psychology of childbirth and I'm almost ashamed that it has taken 20 years to investigate further. The mother's body will tell her what to do – if she is able to hear its instructions and if she is in a physical and mental position to follow them.

Midwifery evidence

Many midwives talk of women's instinctive behaviour during birth, moving around, shifting the pelvis from side to side with rocking movements. In a chapter on mobility and posture in labour, Denis Walsh (2007) writes, 'If you ask observers of nonmedicated labour and births what strikes them most about women's behaviours they will often comment on the labouring woman's apparent inherent restlessness'. It would be all but impossible to analyse this kind of behaviour in a way that would enable it to be used in a Cochrane review. Nevertheless, I believe that instinctive movement can play a huge role in birth. But instinct can operate only when women are free to act on their instincts and this is particularly difficult in the hospital environment, an unfamiliar place with unfamiliar people and unfamiliar rules of behaviour. Too much energy must be spent on dealing with a new social situation at the same time as dealing with the new uncomfortable sensations of the strong contractions of labour. In hospital, all too often those sensations are labelled as 'pain' and women are told that it will only get worse and she should consider an epidural straight away.

Coping with pain or reducing pain?

I believe that there is a distinction to be made between strong, very uncomfortable, *productive* contractions and intrinsically painful *unproductive* contractions, and again I can speak from personal experience and by reading countless birth stories. Buhimschi *et al* (2003) calculate that between 80 and 160 contractions are needed to expel a baby. Out of four labours (i.e. out of between 320 and 640 contractions in total) I had two excruciatingly painful contractions while lying on my side on the bed in an attempt to rest or take a break during the birth of my first child. This was a 'back to back' labour and I had spent the rest of labour sitting bolt upright on the edge of the bed. In the upright position, contractions were very strong and very uncomfortable but bearable (I dreaded another one coming and was glad when it was over but I could cope with them). Having experienced those two painful contractions, I can understand why someone would choose an epidural if they thought all contractions were going to be that painful.

The strength and discomfort of each individual contraction may be an indication of its productivity; I believe that excessive pain is an indication of its lack of productivity. Labour pains have been compared to menstrual cramps but I think menstrual cramps are worse because they are not working against a solid object. Similarly, after-pains, which come after the birth and during the very early days of breastfeeding, are more painful than labour contractions.

In the latent stage of labour, before the cervix has started to open, I believe that painful contractions are a signal to the mother to shift around to let her baby find the best way into the pelvis. It seems that women can distinguish between contractions which are 'doing something' and contractions which are not. If the evolutionary purpose of pain in early labour is to teach the woman that she can do something to alleviate it, insisting that mothers restrict their movement to allow CTG leads to remain in place is downright cruel and counterproductive to efficient labour. Women do protest loudly against the restriction of movement required by continuous monitoring in labour; most birth stories that women tell of good labours contain much information on positions adopted and the quality of contractions.

Further research

There is virtually no research interest in the subjective quality of contractions, their perceived 'productivity' and painfulness. Why is it that some women experience virtually no pain until the baby is almost ready to be born? Their uterus must have been contracting for the cervix to have opened and yet contractions have never crossed over the threshold into consciousness. Is this because the baby is already ideally placed to find his way through the pelvis and the uterus has no need to 'ask the mother to shift position' to help him change his orientation? We need more research like that of Méndez-Bauer which looks at women in normal labour and asks them to report on their pain and comfort. Recording the strength and frequency of contractions alone may satisfy the scientists' need for objectivity, but listening to women would add a rich layer of information that could be used to gain a far better understanding of how the uterus works in labour.

The baby's movements

So much for the mother's movement in labour, what about her baby? The uterus contains another body which can also move. The baby's body is not just a passive object to be moved down the birth canal. There is an optimal position for him to adopt to start his journey through the pelvis, and the best position is head first backwards, 'looking' towards his mother's lower spine. He does not move straight downwards; there is an optimum angle of entry into the pelvis, known as the 'drive angle'. Imagine a balloon – the neck of the balloon, the cervix, is in a more or less fixed position in the pelvis but the main body of the uterus is supported only by the soft tissues of the abdominal wall and has much more movement. The body of the uterus and the neck of the uterus need to line up to enable the baby to have a clear passage through the pelvis. The uterus needs to point the top of his head towards the coccyx, the lowest part of the spine. The uterus is a soft tissue organ, and has to achieve a seamless join with the bony part of the birth canal.

Thus the baby plays an active role in labour even before he starts to move through the pelvis. Babies are born with a set of reflexes, some of which are present only around the time of birth. Reflexes are automatic movements hard wired into the brain; if the nerves on one part of the body are stimulated, another part of the body moves. They are used by paediatricians to assess the neurological condition of the baby at birth but they evolved long before doctors could use them for clinical test purposes. Milani-Comparetti, a paediatric

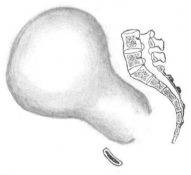

Figure 23: The cervix fits nicely into the pelvis. The balloon is the concept of the drive angle.

neurologist, hypothesised that some of these reflexes evolved to facilitate birth itself (1981). He is convinced that four of the reflexes serve a purpose for birth: the stepping reflex, the Moro reflex, the asymmetric tonic neck reflex and the tonic labyrinthine reflex. (A midwife friend, Joy Horner, and I think that the rooting reflex and the Galant reflex may also play a part.)

Milani-Comparetti postulates that during pregnancy these reflexes allow the fetus to: move around and find the physiologic presentation by searching for the 'invitation of softness' of the pelvic inlet into which he pushes his head with alternating rotations. He suggests that the propulsion pattern is used for fetal collaboration in labour. He was aware of the implications for labour and added that cerebral palsy, which is often characterised by the absence of some neonatal reflexes, may be a *cause* rather than a *consequence* of dysfunctional labour. Being a paediatric neurologist, Milani-Comparetti was an expert in both neonatal reflexes and babies with cerebral palsy. This information should have been picked up by medical defence lawyers. There is a widespread belief that cerebral palsy is caused by lack of oxygen (hypoxia) during labour and, since cerebral palsy leads to the highest legal settlements in obstetric litigation, fear of hypoxia in birth leads to much intervention in childbirth.

Cerebral palsy is a disorder of movement. The incidence of cerebral palsy has remained constant at around two per thousand births for the past 50 years, despite increased fetal monitoring and increased caesarean section. Cerebral palsy may cause difficult labour because, lacking reflexes, the baby is unable to play his full role in finding his way out of the uterus. The irony is that monitoring for signs of fetal hypoxia requires women to be supine, which decreases blood supply to the placenta and may help cause some of the very damage doctors are trying to prevent.

Reflex	Stimulus	Response
Stepping reflex	Held upright with feet touching the ground	Walking motions with legs and feet
Moro reflex	Allow the head to fall back an inch	Arms and legs first extend then pull back towards the body
Asymmetric tonic neck reflex	Turning the head to one side	As the head is turned, the arm and leg on the same side will extend, while the opposite limbs bend.
Tonic labyrinthine reflex	Lying on the back, tilting the head back	The back stiffens and can even arch backwards, the legs straighten, stiffen and push together, toes point, arms bend at the elbows and wrists, and the hands make fists
Galant reflex	Stroking along one side of the spine	Trunk and hips move toward the side of the stimulus
Rooting reflex	Stroking the baby's cheek	Turns head towards the stimulus

Table 1: The reflexes of newly born babies.

The table above shows reflexes that seem to be involved in birth. Milani-Comparetti thought that these hardwired reflexes could help the fetus first to guide himself into the ideal position for entering the birth canal (the invitation to softness) and then to work his way down towards the exit. They should perhaps be renamed fetal reflexes. Some of them disappear after birth because they are no longer needed. I am going to take Milani-Comparetti's word for it that these reflexes are important in birth and look forward to seeing videos showing the mechanisms.

Pas de deux

If labour is a *pas de deux* between the bodies of the mother and her fetus, then we would expect problems if one of the dancing partners is paralysed or rendered immobile. The mother may be immobilised by the bed or encouraged to be still so as not to dislodge the transducers measuring her contractions and her baby's heart rate. The belts holding the transducers may be tight and restrict fetal movement. The lower half of the mother's body may be paralysed by epidural anaesthesia. Systematic reviews and NICE guidelines acknowledge that epidural anaesthesia lengthens labour and that fetal monitoring is associated with a higher rate of surgical delivery. Labour is longer and harder in these circumstances – is it because the movements of the mother and her baby are restricted?

Successful labour and birth is not a question of moving a passive object down the birth canal. The baby moves. Drugs given to the mother may make him sleepy and less active. Sometimes he may be partially paralysed by cerebral palsy with some of those fetal reflexes missing and, sadly, it is well known that labour is harder for mothers who are labouring with a fetus who has already died.

My working hypothesis is that labour will be more efficient and effective when mother and baby are both active and free to move – that is when the mother can voluntarily move her body by working with instinctive cues (including pain), and the fetus can move inside the mother's body by using hard-wired fetal/neonatal reflexes. When people are physically uncomfortable they shift their bodies around until they find a more comfortable position; why should it be any different for the mother and baby during labour?

If you imagine the uterus as a balloon inside the mother's body, both bodies can exert pressure on it, the baby from the inside, the mother's skeleton and other 'hard parts' from the outside (the 'hard parts' being abdominal and skeletal muscles, bones, bladder and so on). I don't believe that today's obstetricians and physiologists have any idea of the importance of maternal position in labour; I think this is because most research is done on women who are confined to bed, because that makes things easier to measure. If, when researching the physiology of labour, doctors consider that the work of labour is performed by a disembodied uterus and they see the baby as an object to be shifted – a 'passenger', then maternal position would be seen as irrelevant.

The other major force acting on the mother and her uterus

and the baby it is carrying is of course gravity. If the mother is lying on her back all the weight will be directed downwards onto the bed, constraining both her own activity and that of her baby.

The very act of measurement may influence what is being recorded. In science, the term 'observer effect' refers to changes that the act of observation will make on a phenomenon being observed. (Wikipedia cites tyre pressure as a case in point, measuring tyre pressure requires measuring the force of escaping air which changes the pressure.) When monitoring uterine activity during labour, the supine position and the tightness of the monitoring belt may directly constrain fetal movements, and thus alter what it is you are trying to measure.

A very long time ago two obstetricians complained about their peers not appreciating the importance of the role of the uterus in getting the baby into a good position. In a lecture to the Royal Society of Medicine in 1938 Caldwell and Moloy said:

> The lower uterine segment and cervix, while dilating in active labour, serve as a guiding factor during engagement [i.e. fitting the head into the inlet of the pelvis]. Scant reference has been made in recent obstetrical literature to the importance of this factor. Barnes described the principle quite accurately by stating that the anterior aspect of the lower uterine segment acted as a 'valve' or 'inclined plane' directing the head downwards and backward. Parvin and others inferred the mechanism when they spoke of a 'dynamic' axis of descent caused by the soft parts which did not always correspond with the so-called 'static' axis of the pelvis itself.

Lining up the baby for birth

Contractions that can be felt before the cervix has started to dilate can serve no function other than to line up the fetus in the best possible position for leaving the uterus and entering the outside world.

Before labour starts in earnest the cervix is three to four centimetres long with its sides aligned top and bottom. (This is the neck of the balloon.) Towards the end of pregnancy, the hormonal 'knot' is untied. The cervix starts to become thinner and shorter. The inner walls of the softer cervix can now be pushed to the outside, allowing the baby to descend further into the pelvis, to 'engage'. For first-time mothers this happens in the last days of pregnancy. This process is called effacement; on vaginal examination the examiner can feel less and less of a column of cervical tissue, as if the cervix were becoming part of the uterus itself. For first-time mothers effacement tends to happen before the lower end of the cervix dilates much, but effacement and dilatation tend to happen simultaneously for mothers who have given birth before. (Think of it as blowing up the neck of a balloon as well as the body of the balloon. Blowing up a balloon is far harder the first time.) I feel that while this is happening, at whatever time it is happening, whether it is in the last days of pregnancy, or the early part of labour, whether or not the mother can feel her contractions, the uterus is working to position the baby in the best place and at the best angle for birth (head first backwards, 'looking' towards his mother's lower spine).

Doctors can tell how ready a woman is to go into labour by assessing the state of the cervix using the Bishop's score (Bishop, 1964). Some of the elements of that score relate to the baby's position which adds weight to the central hypothesis that contractions in early labour serve to place the baby in the optimal position.

A mother can have an easy, short labour if her baby is already in a good position for birth and she does nothing to alter that situation, i.e. she follows the instinctive pain-avoiding cues of her body. A labour that starts well can be impeded by putting her to bed and restricting her movement, and encouraging her to have an epidural to remove sensations of pain before she even requests it.

Latent labour

Clinicians seem to be rather dismissive of contractions that take place before the cervix has started to dilate; women are warned against coming into hospital too soon – the staff don't know what to 'do' with them. Besides, sending them home again relieves pressure on the labour ward. Albeit accidentally, this policy has benefited countless mothers and babies in terms of dynamic positioning in labour, but one has to wonder what effect forced immobility has on women and their babies where labour has been induced and they can't go home and when the baby is not already in the ideal position. Women whose labours are induced are more likely to be tethered to machines, further reducing their mobility.

The unacknowledged work of latent labour is crucial for a good labour. If the baby is not already in a good position, the uterus will contract in the right places to align him well with the exit, contracting where his reflex movements impinge on its internal surface (see below). This might take hours or even days before clinicians will call it active labour, which can be very discouraging for women – if not to say insulting. Women are sent home 'not in labour' which makes them distrust their own bodies. If women are feeling painful contractions they are feeling painful contractions. Sometimes these contractions do not even show up on a fetal monitor because the transducer recording contractions is in the wrong place to pick them up, not because there are no contractions. Obstetricians and midwives call labour before dilatation 'latent' or 'false' labour (it is called 'prodomal' labour in the USA). 'Active' labour is deemed to have started only when there are regular and painful contractions and the cervix has opened to 4 cm. Women are told that contractions should be getting closer together and stronger. The obstetrician wants to see visual signs of labour, i.e. contractions on a print-out, and to feel cervical dilatation on vaginal examination, i.e. the cervix has opened to about 4 centimetres. This is an arbitrary distinction, largely determined by when caregivers think a mother needs to be admitted to the labour ward. (This somewhat cynical attitude of mine proved justified when the American College of Obstetricians and Gynecologists changed the definition of active labour from 4 cm to 6 cm.) What the woman herself feels is deemed irrelevant. Sometimes, although rarely, mothers reach the pushing stage without becoming aware of any contractions at all – their cervix has opened from 0 to 10 centimetres without them knowing they were in labour – while other women have painful contractions for many hours or even days before the baby is born. Scattered throughout the popular press and birth websites are women's stories of being sent home 'not in labour' or told 'you have hours to go' only for babies to be born unexpectedly quickly on return home, in hospital car parks, or before the midwife has time to put her gloves on. Once the baby is in the optimal position he can be born very quickly. Women can go from 5 centimetres dilated to fully dilated in five minutes. And yet, despite women's reports, the textbooks don't change their own story of what constitutes normal labour. After all, these are the labours that the writers of textbooks never see.

The truth is that every labour is different because there are a myriad ways mother and baby can act and react with each other via the elastic and contractile interface of the uterus and cervix. Unless and until medical scientists start to look at how labour works when women and babies are free to move, they are unlikely to get much further forward in understanding normal birth. It is of little benefit to carry on looking at animal models, even primates, our closest relatives, because for human beings there is such a tight fit between the fetal head and the maternal pelvis that positioning for birth is absolutely the most crucial aspect of uterine function in labour. Only human mothers have to position their large-headed baby to get into the best position to negotiate the human pelvis which contains a 120-degree bend. Only human babies must rotate their way through the pelvis, entering it facing one direction and leaving it in another, pausing to turn again even as they are being born.

As for his journey through the pelvis itself, the baby makes a series of position changes which are known as the cardinal movements. While it is possible for most babies to be born from most starting positions there is an ideal starting position. Think of it as analogous to the starting position a sprinter adopts for a race. He could start facing away from the winning post, he could stand on one leg, he could even stand on his head while waiting for the starting pistol, but to have the best chance of winning the race he uses the starting blocks provided.

6 The science behind the choreography

The complexity of human uterine function and regulation is one of the great wonders of nature and represents a daunting challenge to unravel. (Quote from blurb for *Biomechanics of the Gravid Uterus*. Miftahof RN, Nam HG, 2011.)

Arpad Csapo, a physiologist who devoted his life to understanding how the uterus works, described the mechanics thus: "A community of over 200 billion smooth muscle cells must work in concert to guarantee the safe delivery of the newborn. Any regulatory error that disrupts the synchronic or directional contractility of this community, jeopardises normal parturition and exposes the fetus to grave hazards..." What else is 'smooth muscles must work in concert' and 'directional contractility' but physiological, or biomechanical, choreography?

Unfortunately, the very next sentence reads "Preventive obstetrics, an ever increasing reality in the management of labor, evolved from analytical uterine physiology." (Csapo, 1973). The problem is that preventive obstetrics evolved from a poor understanding of analytical uterine physiology. It is in direct conflict with normal birth because it is virtually blind to one of the two triggers to contraction – the stretch-contract reflex – and it relegates maternal position to a 'nice to have' but non-essential aspect of labour management. As we found in chapter 3, all the clinical guidelines recommend encouraging women to assume upright positions but none realise the vital importance of maternal position. If they did, the obstetric labour room would be organised around the woman's need for comfortable positions in labour not the obstetrician's need for a supine patient and electronic fetal monitoring. Preventive obstetrics has plenty to say and do about supplying the uterus with oxytocin via an intravenous drip, but infusing this artificial hormone may totally override positioning signals from the fetal and maternal bodies.

Biomechanics of position in labour

The biomechanical process which explains how the uterus can 'manipulate' the fetus into the best possible position to start his journey through his mother's pelvis is the stretch-contract reflex. In whatever place it is stretched, the muscle of the uterus reacts by contracting (Wray, 1993); the contraction is initiated in cells at the area where the uterine muscle has been stretched. These cells are known as pacemakers. All uterine cells have the ability to become pacemakers (Buhmischi *et al*, 2003). Textbooks still maintain that pacemakers are located at either side of the uterus at the cornua (where the fallopian tubes meet the uterus) but there is little evidence for a fixed pacemaker area in the uterine muscle: any muscle cell can act as a pacemaker cell and pacemaker cells can change from one contraction to the other (Devedeux, 1993). Contractions may be strongest at the fundus but they do not necessarily originate there. They originate at pacemaker cells which are, according to Buhimschi *et al* (2003): 'autonomously active muscle cells'. They go on to

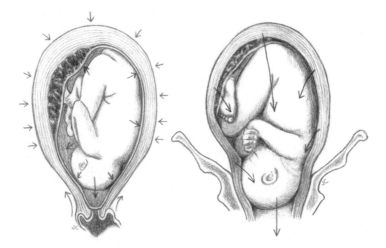

Figure 24: Left: Direction of contractions. Intra-uterine pressure. Early first stage, intact waters, lower segment passive. *Right:* Direction of contractions in the second stage of labour. Direct uterine pressure, full dilatation, membranes ruptured, fetal axis pressure inevitable (after Berkeley and Dupuy, 1932).

state that 'all myometrial [uterine muscle] cells are potential pacemakers and can assume the role from one contraction to the next ... A characteristic of myometrial cells is that they can either be excited by action potentials (pace-follower cells) or generate electrical activity themselves (pace-maker cells)'.

This is not what obstetricians and midwives are taught. The current view, known as 'fundal dominance', states that contractions start at the top of the uterus, at the side where a hypothetical 'pacemaker' is situated, and work their way down towards the cervix, pulling up cervical tissue to open the cervix. Thus, the classical theory sees the task of opening the cervix as the most important function of the contractions of labour. Active labour is deemed not even to have started until there is cervical dilatation. This view of the activity of the uterus has dominated obstetric thinking since the 1950s when it was first proposed. The reality is that women can experience contractions for many hours or even days before they are said to be in labour and even the textbooks admit that the onset of labour is difficult to define, and that there is a continuum of uterine activity which eventually evolves into active labour.

If one forgets the cervix for a moment and instead considers that the ultimate purpose of labour is to give birth, then the contractions of latent, early or prodomal labour, if not opening the cervix, must be doing something else, and what else is there to do other than to position the baby in the right place to start his journey? I remember many times during pregnancy lying in the bath watching my baby moving around inside me (reacting to the hot water?) only for him to be folded back into the fetal position. The fetal position is also the shape of the uterus. The elastic uterus enfolds and contains the fetus. During pregnancy this activity could be a passive reaction, merely the result of the natural elasticity of the uterus, but during labour the uterus contracts and hardens periodically. Could it be that the uterus is working to position the fetus in the ideal place to exit? Could excessively painful contractions result from the failure of the uterus to achieve this objective? If so, why is it failing? Could it be that even the most powerful muscle in the body is unable to cope with a bony obstruction? If the uterus is unable to overcome the resistance of bone, then the only solution is to move the bone by moving the mother. Once you can see this, it becomes almost unthinkable to immobilise a woman in bed and anaesthetise her pain. You would do your utmost to enable her to shift around and make every contraction count.

A book such as this is not the right place to propose such a radical change to obstetric scientific thinking but I have no other option. What I have done is to draw together numerous different threads in the scientific literature, combine them with evidence from women's experience, look at the clinical evidence of outcomes for women whose babies are lying in awkward positions, look at the outcomes of women labouring in places where they can move freely (by and large, at home and in birth centres) and where they can't (by and large, in obstetric units) and build an outline of what I think may be happening. Presenting a bullet-proof scientific case would probably take another 20 years and, the politics of science being what it is, such research would be unlikely to attract funding even if a research institution would be prepared to take it on. After 40 years of trying, Elaine Morgan's aquatic ape hypothesis is still very much on the fringes of the scientific establishment's view of human evolution, largely because it is almost impossible to dislodge establishment thinking that mankind evolved on the African savannah. Too many influential people still have too much to lose.

The aquatic ape hypothesis has few practical implications for modern life but how we care for women in labour is crucial. Seeing film footage of yet another woman lying in bed, whether in agony or having her pain anaesthetised by epidural, tethered to machines and ending up with a caesarean section, is enough to make me want to do something to change the way our society manages birth. I can see absolutely no harm in trying to change the way people think about the mother's and baby's physical positions in labour and how they may interact with each other. The whole of western obstetrics has practically ignored the concept of maternal and fetal positioning. What chance have I as a lay person to change anything except by enlisting the help of anyone and everyone who agrees that it is time to change our thinking about birth?

I have come to this notion largely through intuition. Think of it as the beginning of a jigsaw puzzle. I caught a fleeting glimpse of the picture on the box 27 years ago and since then have come across little to refute it and much to support it. The puzzle pieces have been slowly dropping into place. To go back over that whole process would take too much space in this book and many more years' work, time for another generation of women to have their labours managed according to the current theory. I think it's worth asking other people to help put some more pieces into the puzzle. The puzzle is there for the solving.

Problems with the current view

The problem with the fundal dominance theory is that it sees the uterus as a battering ram (the powers) forcing open the door of the birth canal (the passage) and pushing a passive object (the passenger) through it. Unfortunately this rather violent view of birth came at a time when oxytocin had been synthesised by pharmacologists and Syntocinon (known as Pitocin in the US) could be produced in large quantities for clinical use. Thus obstetricians tended to see only one solution to problems in labour: increase the power of the battering ram by infusing increasing amounts of artificial oxytocin until the battering ram did its work. The fact that this solution to problems in labour does produce clinical results in terms of speeding up labour reinforced the belief in fundal dominance. It also reinforced doctors' belief that they could control labour but at the same time it sapped women's confidence that their bodies were capable of giving birth. Hospital midwives were perhaps stuck somewhere in the middle. They could see that some women could give birth without artificial oxytocin but they were also the ones who administered the drug and they could see its effects. The controversy about the overuse of artificial oxytocin continues into this century.

The origin of the current view is found in the work of Samuel Reynolds in the 1950s. He strapped six uterine strain gauge transducers onto the abdomen of a woman in labour and inserted a balloon pressure monitoring device into her uterus. Seven graphs were plotted simultaneously showing the activity at all seven sites: six showed surface activity above the uterus and one showed the overall internal pressure. In normal, straightforward labour, traditional stretch transducers seemed to demonstrate a descending gradient of contraction intensity, with the two transducers at mid-uterus recording simultaneous but less intense contractions than the two at the fundus, and with the two transducers placed on the lower segment recording a flat line. There was often more activity on one side of the uterus than the other. Together, these findings seemed to imply that there was a pacemaker at the top of the uterus at one side or the other and that contractions spread downwards, weakening as they went. Fundal pressure was opening the cervix and pushing the baby out in one easy action. This is one set of traces I'm not going to reproduce. They had a simplicity and elegance to them that seemed to provide utterly compelling visual evidence for the current theory. The traces had a ring of truth about them and were utterly seductive. As soon as I found one of Reynolds' papers (Reynolds, 1951) I wasted countless hours fitting its implications around my own model of the balloon – only to find at the eleventh hour that the pattern was an illusion.

Even at the time the current fundal dominance theory was disputed. Mylks *et al* (1954) built a latex balloon model

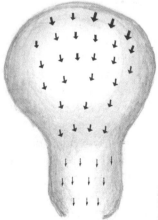

Figure 25: The current view: Direction of contractions according to Reynolds, 1949.

of a uterus and overlaid it with thicknesses of towelling to simulate the abdominal wall. He and his colleagues modelled contractions by filling their model uterus with water under different pressures and found a *reverse* gradient of contractions, i.e. changes to the abdominal wall do not necessarily reflect changes at the uterus. This suggested that the downward gradient was likely to be an artefact of the measurement system. The top of the uterus rises outwards during a contraction. The descending pattern found by Reynolds seems to have been caused by a greater distension to the abdominal wall at the top of the uterus than at the lower segment, i.e. changes to the abdominal wall did not reflect changes at the uterus. The lower end of the uterus cannot move so much because it is more or less fixed inside the pelvis, the middle section rises a little, while the fundus moves furthest because it can. Perhaps all that Reynolds was seeing were contractions strong enough to raise the uterus against the force of gravity and stretch the mother's abdomen. If, in the 1950s, measuring strain at the abdominal wall outside the uterus was not capable of providing any detail about the mechanical activity of the underlying uterus, then the basis for a pacemaker at one side or the other at the fundus, which was hypothesised at that time, loses its theoretical underpinning. Buhimschi's 2003 paper on the forces of labour still gives Reynolds as the reference for 'fundal dominance'; it is about time that the theory was exploded. Electronic fetal monitoring presents midwives with practical difficulties when a mother is labouring in an 'alternative' position. If the mother is leaning forward her abdomen will already be fully stretched and the abdominal transducer would record no strain and so fail to record a contraction. Besides which, transducers tend to fall off. If the lawyers and doctors still require fetal monitoring then they should push for better fetal monitors that will work with the mother labouring in 'alternative' positions.

Nevertheless, the tracing from the fundus of outward displacement *did* usually correlate well with balloon catheter recordings of intrauterine pressure. Strain measurements at the abdominal wall *do often* reflect the total strength of a contraction. External tocography is less invasive than internal pressure monitoring and, although it paints rather a crude picture of contractions, it can be used for monitoring; measuring the extent of displacement of the uterus during a contraction does approximate fairly well to intrauterine pressure. External tocography caught on, technology companies fell over each other to produce fetal monitors, and hospital birth has never been the same since. The combination of synthetic oxytocin and fetal monitoring has been devastating for mothers and babies.

Nagel and Schaldach (1983) pointed out what is to me the worst drawback – the constraints on the mother's movement:

> Even this restricted performance may only be obtained when it is ensured that the transducer remains at its original site throughout the recording period and that the measuring conditions are not changed by the alteration of the patient's position. In very many cases, these requirements cannot be met; indeed, the maintenance of a given position by the patient might even be dangerous for her and the fetus ... Although tocography has become a routine method for the monitoring of uterine contractions, it is not capable of providing information on the detailed mechanical activity of the myometrium [uterine muscle].

Recently, medical physicists have been working towards a greater understanding of how the uterus works in labour by revisiting electromyography, recording electrical activity of the muscle of the uterus (Karlsson, 2007, see ehg.ru.is/Papers/BKarlsson_MEDICON.pdf) and by measuring magnetic fields (La Rosa et al, 2009, see www.ese.wustl.edu/~nehorai/research/ra/MMG3.html). Electromyography picks up the electrical signals of contracting cells. Uterine muscle cell contractions are the end result of electrical activity – the discharging of action potentials – at the muscle cell wall. Individual uterine muscle cells work on the all or nothing principle. Either they fire and contract or they rest. An *action potential* is a short-lasting event in which the electrical membrane potential of a cell rapidly rises and then falls. Action potentials occur in several types of animal cells, called excitable cells, which include neurons and muscle cells. In neurons, they play a central role in cell-to-cell communication. They are the means by which a nervous

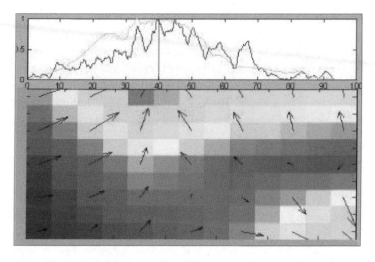

Figure 26: The grid is a snapshot of the electrical activity of the uterus at the peak of a contraction (x-axis 40 seconds into the trace) as calculated from a 4x4 grid of electrodes. The smooth line on the graph was recorded by tocography, the jagged line is the average of electrical activity. The rectangles beneath represent differences in activity between the sites. The arrows represent direction of travel of the strength of electrical activity as a contraction propagates. At the peak of the contraction, most of the activity is directed towards the fundus, not away from it. If the stretch-contract theory is to be believed, there is a pacemaker at the bottom left of the array recorded by the electrodes sited 8 centimetres below the mother's umbilicus.

impulse jumps from nerve cell to nerve cell. Once the uterus has been 'wired up' for labour, turning it into a functional network, action potentials play a similar role in the uterus. Action potentials also activate intracellular processes. In muscle cells, for example, an action potential is the first step in a very quick chain of events which leads to contraction. Early in pregnancy, the poor electrical coupling among the cells is responsible for the quiescent status of the uterus. Contractions happen all over the place all the time but they do not spread because there are few electrical connections with adjacent cells. As delivery approaches, rising oestrogen levels lead to the synthesis of connexin-43 to allow the propagation of electrical activity from cell to cell. Eventually the sheer number of these connections allows contractions to spread further and further and to be capable of inducing progressive cervical dilatation and downwards pressure. The uterus acts holistically.

Before labour, if the uterus is responding to being stretched, only the stretched portion contracts. Once the billions of muscle cells at the uterus have been organised into a network of connected cells, the contractions can spread out in a wave from the stretched portion. It is the propagation of electrical activity at the uterus that leads to the coordinated and effective contractions of labour. I believe that the electrical signals now picked up by electromyography and labelled as 'pacemakers' will be found to originate at places where the uterus has been stretched – perhaps the area where the baby is kicking.

The images obtained through electromyography do not support the current view of contractions starting from the top and working their way down but do seem to show the presence of pacemaker activity elsewhere in the uterus, with the site of initiation changing from snapshot to snapshot. Both these papers are linked to images showing the mother lying on her back and lack any indication of the lie of the baby in the uterus, but electromyography does hold out some hope. Electromyography coupled with information about fetal position could cast more light on this matter. It could also measure the effects of changing the mother's position. Theoretically, it would be possible to test the hypothesis that labour is a working partnership between the baby and his mother's uterus by building a computer model which includes the baby and predicts pacemaker sites according to known fetal reflexes.

Understanding more about monitoring has cleared up something that had long been bothering me; if the uterus is contracting, i.e. getting *smaller*, why do monitors measure an *increase* in strain during a contraction? This mystery is cleared up by the knowledge that what is being measured is the stretch of the abdominal wall rather than the contraction of the uterus.

Going into labour – the transforming uterus

In 2015 I came across a snippet of information that led me on a whole new journey of thinking about mechanisms which could tip women into labour (Mesiano et al 2015 in: Knobil and Neill's, Physiology of Reproduction, 2015). The information concerned genetic differences between chimpanzees (with whom we share 99% of our genes) and humans. One of the biggest differences in genes concerning reproduction is changes in a class of biochemicals that I hadn't encountered before – matrix metalloproteins MMPs. MMPs (collagenases) break down collagen, the stiffening agent in the cervix, into a watery substance (see page 76). This is important because collagen makes the cervix stretch resistant and may be what helps to maintain pregnancy and prevent premature labour. I also struggled through a book entitled *Biomechanics of the Gravid Human Uterus* in which biophysicists have constructed a model of how the uterus works in labour using the laws of physics (e.g. force and elasticity). (The equations were beyond me but my knowledge of biomechanics improved.)

I learnt about the substance in which non-skeletal muscle cells are embedded, which is known as the extra cellular matrix (ECM). All smooth muscle organs such as the heart and the uterus need some sort of structural scaffolding. Muscle alone is too floppy to maintain shape without collagen.

It came as a revelation to find that the cervix was not the only structure to contain collagen. Uterine muscle is also constrained in a scaffolding of collagen, not so stiff as the cervix perhaps, but scaffolding all the same, which stiffens the tissue and therefore limits available stretch of the uterine wall. Imagine a balloon blown up inside a grocery net, the net stops full inflation of the balloon; it constricts the amount of achievable stretch.

I wondered whether, like the cervix, the uterus also undergoes structural change before labour can take off in earnest. During pregnancy, the uterus merely folds back the kicking fetus back to fetal position. During labour, loss of collagen scaffolding enables the fetus to stretch and trigger contraction in a greater area of the uterine wall.

The physical effect of collagen breakdown would be to transform the biomechanical properties of the uterus, making it less rigid and more elastic. If it can stretch more, then it can contract more. A pregnant uterus could be transformed into a labouring uterus simply by breaking down some of the collagen. Loss of collagen flips the uterus into labouring mode. Now when the baby kicks, a larger portion of the uterus would be affected and the muscle of the uterus would react and contract over a larger area. The more the scaffolding was broken down, the more the uterus could contract and the stronger contractions would become. Taken in conjunction with the increase in contraction promoting hormones and the increased electrical network connections at term the full power of the uterus is unleashed.

This model reflects what we know happens towards the end of pregnancy (from about 36 weeks) and during labour itself. The movements of the baby would then have more and more effect on the activity of the uterus, the baby moves himself out of his incubator as it is transformed into an ejector seat. But this process must take place over time and there must be mechanisms in

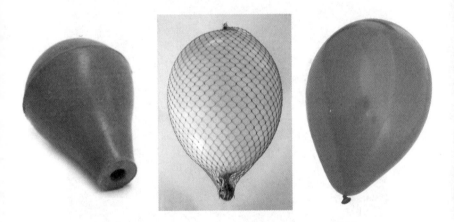

Figure 27: Picture the difference between the behaviour of these three items when you press a couple of fingers into them: If you press the rubber bulb it will make a dent in the rubber and then spring back. If you press a party balloon in a net, the net stops you pressing very far in. Free the balloon from the constraints of the net and imagine a baby inside with its head acting as a stopper (instead of the knot). Now any pressure you exert will move the baby downwards. Try it yourself, partially blow up a balloon, insert a ping pong ball and experiment. (See it here: www.youtube.com/watch?v=URyEZusnjBI or search for YouTube balloon labour)

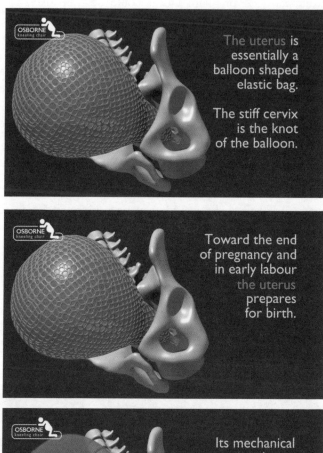

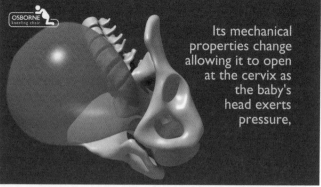

Figure 28: As the balloon of the uterus gradually loses its scaffolding of collagen, fetal movements will cause stronger contractions that spread further. The pressure of the baby's head opens the cervix to become contiguous with the birth canal (from www.youtube.com/watch?v=JIHHH32US3g).

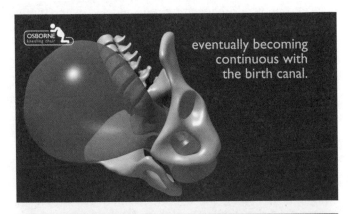

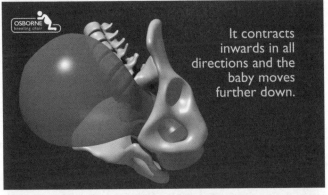

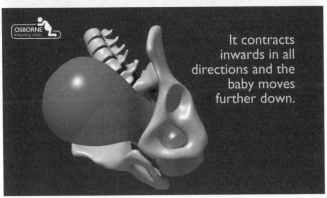

Figure 28 continued: You have to imagine the baby for now. Usually, the back of his head will be behind the symphysis pubis, his face fitting into the sacrum at the back of the pelvis. Forward leaning lets gravity play its part in the work of birth.

place to prevent it happening too suddenly, when the mother doesn't perceive herself to be in a safe place. She retains some hormonal control and the reason why hypnobirthing has been found to be so effective is because it changes her mental state and therefore her secretion of labour stopping hormones. The model explains why the uterus is more prone to rupture during induction of labour by oxytocin: if it hasn't yet had time to lose its collagen scaffolding it will not have the ability to stretch and may rupture instead.

I offered this possible mechanism for the onset of labour to the *British Journal of Obstetrics and Gynaecology* and they thought enough of the idea to respond by offering me the chance to participate in a debate (Jowitt, 2018), which ended up being about whether freedom of maternal movement is more important than electronic fetal monitoring (you can guess which side of the argument I opted for!).

There is evidence that the collagen content of the uterus sampled at caesarean section is higher at pre-labour elective caesarean section than at in-labour caesarean section (Morrione, 1962) and evidence that the enzyme which breaks down collagen, collagenase, increases during labour (Osmers et al, 1994). Prostaglandins break down collagen in the uterus (Chiossi et al, 2012) Winkler et al (1999) found that collagen breaks down during labour. It seems that labour does involve breaking down the collagen scaffolding which makes it more elastic so that fetal movements stretching it will have progressively more effect. We know that the uterus quickly reduces in size after birth (involution) so the only novel part of my theory is that a change of substance may start *before* labour and so help initiate labour and may be responsible for the increasingly powerful of contractions of labour. We know that Braxton Hicks contractions start to happen about four weeks before the birth.

There has been a deafening silence from physiologists in the UK but a US obstetrician who is interested in how the uterus functions as a whole organ (i.e. not just looking at what happens at the biochemical and hormonal level, but how the biomechanics may be affected) is interested in the concepts I have outlined and thinks that stretch may play a role in allowing labour contractions to involve the whole uterine muscle network, a process which he terms mechanotransduction (Young, 2018: this paper would be a useful introduction to anyone wanting a more technical introduction to the biomechanics of uterine function.) Young considers that the extended electrical network alone is not enough to account for the involvement of the whole body of the uterus in the contractions of labour.

I wondered why no one had noticed this before and have come to the conclusion firstly that physiologists have become so specialised in analysing biochemicals that they fail to consider the gross physical effects on the tissue they are studying (in this case the link between elasticity, stretch and contraction) and, secondly, that even if they do, no one seems to consider the baby as a possible cause of stretching the uterus and thereby initiating contractions.

We need mother and baby centred physiology instead of merely thinking in terms of the 'powers' and the 'passenger' (see page 80) and thereby ignoring the activity of the baby and his mother.

Evidence for the dynamic uterus

This theory is speculative. Had it been generally known in obstetric circles then I would have to conclude that the entire profession is a conspiracy against womankind, which I don't think is the case. Instead there is collective blindness to normal physiology. However, we do now have the means of enlightenment.

Even if there is no permanent pacemaker at the fundus, the top of the uterus, there is no doubt that the force of contractions opens the cervix in labour; this activity is inherent in the mechanical properties of any balloon. A party balloon has no pacemaker – blow one up, leave it unknotted, let it go, and see which way it flies. The escaping air is always going to propel it forwards. Once the uterus has changed from a closed system, with a hormonal 'knot' keeping it shut, to an open system with an opening cervix, wherever they start, contractions are bound to exert pressure towards the cervix, the site of least resistance.

How does the stretch-contract reflex work?

Stretching uterine muscle leads to the secretion and release of prostaglandins which are biochemical substances already available or quickly manufactured and released locally (Horton *et al*, 1971; Poyser *et al*, 1971; Manabe *et al*, 1983). Wikipedia puts it thus: 'prostaglandins are mediators and have a variety of strong physiological effects, such as regulating the contraction and relaxation of smooth muscle tissue. Prostaglandins … differ from hormones in that they are not produced at a discrete site but in many places throughout the human body. Also, their target cells are present in the immediate vicinity of the site of their secretion (of which there are many). Amongst other functions, prostaglandins sensitize spinal neurons to pain and induce labor.'

The common link connecting various types of prostaglandin release is distortion or damage of cell membranes (Piper 1973). Distortion is stretch.

The links between prostaglandins, stretch, contraction and pain are the key to understanding the reason why maternal position may be so important for a good labour. There are two stimuli to their production, firstly stretch and secondly oxytocin. According to Buhimschi *et al* (2003) the two stimuli have an equal effect. Both release prostaglandins.

I believe that the stretch-contract reflex is by far the most important thing to consider as far as normal birth is concerned. Poor maternal positioning – the dominance of the bed, the consequent supine position and the abolition of pain cues with epidural anaesthesia – may be preventing the stretch-contract reflexes from allowing the choreography of labour to unfold as nature intended. If the mother is unable to move or shift her position and the contraction does not move the fetus, then the same area of the uterus will undergo repeated stimulation by stretch, more prostaglandin will be secreted and more pain will be felt. There may even come a time when the reserves of prostaglandin and calcium (the fuel of muscle contraction) are exhausted and labour stalls completely. The obstetric solution to dysfunctional labour – artificial oxytocin infusion – bombards the uterus with unphysiological amounts of oxytocin, over-riding and bypassing the directional cues that would come from the stretch-contract reflex driven by the fetal body. If so, it is no wonder that caesarean section is such a common outcome of labours driven by artificial oxytocin. Forceps and ventouse deliveries will also be more necessary as the baby is driven through the cervix in a less than optimal position.

Uncoordinated contractions

Midwives and obstetricians are taught that contractions can be uncoordinated and that such contractions are painful and fail to open the cervix. The very concept of uncoordinated contractions, which seem to be well established as a cause of abnormal labour, makes sense only if they *can* start from different places – and perhaps at more than one place at a time. If, rather than being merely labelled 'uncoordinated', these contractions were to be seen as positioning contractions, their purpose becomes clear. If the work of contractions before complete dilatation is to position the baby for birth (which does seem logical) then repeated ineffective contractions will be the result of repeated failed attempts of the baby to reposition himself. Why should these attempts fail? If the mother is lying on her back, the uterus may be constrained by the barrier of her spine or internal organs. The baby may be physically unable to stretch the area that needs to be stretched for him to progress.

It is now possible to see a printout of uncoordinated contractions. The scientists found contraction patterns to be surprisingly complex:

> It is possible at times to observe ascendant activation patterns while for the majority of the contractions the activation patterns is descendant. In this situation, the uterine activity begins at the lower electrodes or those situated on one side and then propagate to the other electrodes. Several origins of the activity could often be observed. (Karlsson et al, 2007)

There is much obstetric language that already contains hints about the importance of positioning. Before the head becomes engaged, it is said to be 'floating'. Obstetricians generally use this term to describe the baby's position in terms of the bones of the pelvis (see the next chapter) but it will also be 'floating' in the amniotic fluid and 'floating' implies that it still has room to move. Early and first stage labour are not just a question of the baby moving downwards to become engaged but of rotating the axis of his body so that the most optimal diameter of his head engages in the best position to pass through the pelvis. Stronger contractions at the middle of the uterus will push the baby inwards rather than downwards and may well serve to position him more centrally within the uterus and place his head directly above the cervix so that it can become 'well applied' to the cervix, another obstetric term explicitly concerning position. The clinical evidence and theory stated in the clinical literature for upright position is that labour goes better when the fetal head is 'closely applied' to the cervix. When the fetal head is closely applied to the cervix it is stretching it equally in all directions and sending a stronger uniform upward signal.

As the next chapter will attempt to show, the baby needs to enter the pelvis at an angle which will give him the least constricted pathway through the tunnel of the pelvis. Fetal reflexes steer him and position him (looking for Milani-Comparetti's 'invitation to softness') down into the pelvis and onto the cervix, using the stretch-contract mechanism of the uterus.

The onset of labour is gradual; as midwives put it a woman can be 'niggling' for days before labour gets going in earnest. (Is labour 'niggling' the fetus wriggling?) It can be very frustrating not knowing quite when labour has started and whether the contractions will progress into full-blown labour. Women can have contractions at night which then stop the following morning. Night-time contractions which fade away in the morning reflect the effect of circadian rhythms of oxytocin secretion – in primates more oxytocin is secreted in the hours of darkness when stress hormone levels are low (Honnebier, 1989). Although such contractions are a sign that the uterus has been 'wired up' for labour, until the collagen matrix at the cervix has broken down, the body won't tip over into full labour. Labour can't get started in earnest until the cervix can open. Labour operates on a positive feedback mechanism which itself is held in check by the stress hormone systems which operate under circadian rhythms (Jowitt, 1993).

Latent labour

I believe that the mother and baby both need the freedom to move in the early stages of labour before the baby is ideally positioned for the journey through the pelvis. If the mother is stuck in one position on a bed, she may be tensing up her abdominal muscles as a reaction to pain and creating another 'wall' preventing her baby from stretching her uterus in the place he needs it to contract to give him the chance to wriggle his way around. I think this is where pathological pain can be differentiated from the 'normal' sensations of contractions and, if the mother doesn't attempt to change her position, her baby may be unable to move to a better position. The baby may well make repeated attempts to shift his position to no avail, the same portion of uterus may receive repeated stimulation and yet nothing can change because there are physical barriers. This is the pain that should be a signal to the mother to change her position and find a comfortable position to reduce the sensation of pain. I feel that a comfortable position is one which will

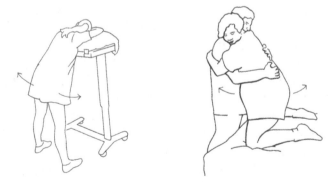

Figure 29: Forward leaning positions: *Standing, swaying with a tray table* and *Kneeling, rocking with partner support.*

allow the uterus to be stretched wherever the baby 'wants' to stretch it, and it seems to me that the forward-leaning position gives the uterus the most freedom from external constraints. Even in programmes such as *One Born Every Minute* one sees mothers leaning forward, supported by their partner. *The Labor Progress Handbook*, by Penny Simkin and Ruth Ancheta, has numerous illustrations of forward-leaning positions which Penny recommends for labours where the baby is not in the best position. Forward leaning certainly worked in my two easiest labours. Penny Simkin talks about progressing and non-progressing contractions and obstetricians refer to 'false labour' and 'active labour', but there is nothing false about the uterus steering the baby to the best position. I prefer positioning and propulsive contractions.

Pressure is evenly distributed in the uterus during pregnancy when the uterus is closed. However, after the system becomes open at the beginning of labour (when the 'knot' at the cervix is untied) there will be no upward pressure from the cervix, only pressure towards the exit.

Oxytocin is not released into the bloodstream in large quantities until the second stage of labour. Throughout the first stage, while the baby is still contained within the uterus, it looks as if the primary stimulus for contraction is stretch. However, once the baby has started to pass out of the uterus he loses most of his ability to stretch it, although he does now have the space to kick against the fundus. Think of the uterus now as a floppy balloon, starting to go down as its contents are expelled.

There is often a natural break in contractions at this point in normal labour. In the absence of stretch at the uterus, another stimulus for contraction is needed and it comes from pressure on the internal part of the clitoris which leads to a surge of natural oxytocin – Ferguson's reflex (See below 'The clitoris').

Researchers studied the effects of maternal position on the strength of contractions and length of labour and found that upright positions are associated with stronger contractions and shorter labour (Caldeyro-Barcia 1950). One mechanism behind this may be that the drive angle is better and the fetal head is better applied to the cervix. An optimal drive angle allows the

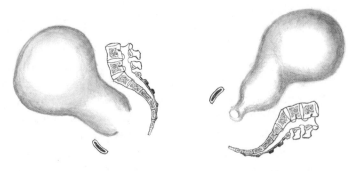

Figure 30: The cervix is suspended by the cervical ligaments in the mid pelvis. Lying supine compromises the drive angle. (Concept figure not to scale.)

uterus to retain its symmetrical pear shape even when the fetal head has descended into the birth canal (see Figure 30). A drive angle which aligns the fetal head squarely with the cervix will allow a more even pressure on the cervix. The drive angle needs to be optimised for effective contractions but is also very important for the passage through the pelvis as we shall see in the next chapter. Even as I write, more pieces of the puzzle are dropping into place; could it be that a suboptimal drive angle is responsible for much of the pain of labour? Janie McCoy King (1993), another mother like me with no clinical expertise who also developed an interest in these matters in the 1990s, describes a physical manoeuvre which can help labours which have stalled – the mother lifts her own abdomen up to change the drive angle. This can be so effective that she warns mothers to try it only once they are in the place where they intend to give birth. It is picked up by Penny Simkin (a childbirth educator and doula who trained as a physiotherapist) and her colleague Ruth Ancheta in their book *The Labor Progress Handbook*.

The clitoris

Since the first edition of this book I discovered that, like an iceberg, most of the clitoris is hidden away out of sight. Rather than being merely a small protrusion at the top of the pubic arch, it is 10 cm long. It consists of a main body which is mostly hidden away along the symphysis pubis at the front of the pelvis, but which tunnels through to the outside at the apex of the pubic arch where it is visible. It also has two legs (the crura) which attach to the sides of the pubic arch and two bulbs (also known as the vestibular bulbs) which extend slightly backwards and surround the vagina. The main function of the clitoris has been totally missed by anatomists. The commonly accepted function is to give the female sexual pleasure but in this it fails; vaginal orgasm is relatively rare. Humans mate face-to-face instead of the male mounting the female from behind. Other primates have penile bones which allow internal stimulation but man enters at a different angle and no longer has a stiff enough member to stimulate the internal clitoris. However, situated where it is, at the baby's exit from his mother's body, it seems sensible to consider that the clitoris may well have a role to play in birth. If this is the case (and, after all, the birth process must be a far stronger driver of evolution than female sexual pleasure) that role has to be activation of the fetal ejection reflex. Again the stimulus is activated by part of the fetal body, in this case the back of his head, as it passes through the pelvis. The baby's head impinges on 8,000 nerve endings and a message is sent to the

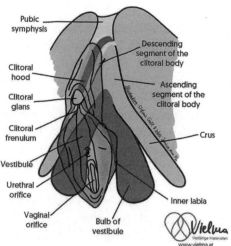

Figure 31: Most of the clitoris is hidden inside. The main body is at the front of the pelvis adjacent to the symphysis pubis (Illustration Stefanie Grübl).

hypothalamus, the so-called heart of the brain (Leng, 2018), to deliver 'lots of oxytocin and quickly'. At the same time the clitoris becomes engorged, providing cushions of blood-filled tissue to protect the baby's head as he is born. Birth is orgasmic. Fluttering vaginal contractions help the process.

Trying to get the picture

I have found that extending the balloon analogy into a hypothetical three-dimensional hollow trampoline helps me get an intuitive understanding of the forces of labour. After all the uterus is a network of elastic fibres. I groped towards an understanding of the biomechanics of the uterus in my previous book many years ago with pictures of how, in a standard trampoline, the elastic forces direct the trampolinist back into the centre. I even showed what might happen if there was a rigid pole beneath the trampoline (an analogy for the mother's spine) but, apart from learning that the uterus works using a stretch-contract mechanism, I failed to find much evidence to support these ideas. Twenty years later there is so much more evidence.

Figures 32 and 33 were drawn to illustrate the nucleus of a radium atom (it is an axially symmetric octupole!) but it is also a very good approximation for the network of muscle of

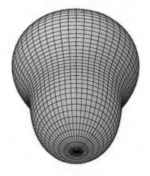

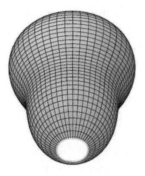

Figure 32: Imagine the uterus as a three-dimensional trampoline. If the 'knot' is tied contractions fold the fetus into the middle.

Figure 33: Once the 'knot' starts to untie contractions will work the fetus downwards.

the uterus at the end of pregnancy. All it lacks is the cervix itself. Moreover, it illustrates an optimal drive angle if you visualise it inside a pregnant woman standing with her back to you. The top part is spherical. The lower end, known as the lower segment, is thinner and contains more fibrous tissue but less muscle. The lower segment has developed and elongated in the second half of pregnancy and contains the baby's head when he is presenting head first. Like the cervix, it stretches to accommodate the descending fetal head, in fact the top end of the cervix almost becomes part of the lower segment as it effaces and opens.

All the lines on the 'trampoline' represent strings of elastic muscle fibres (40 billion muscle cells organised into longitudinal, spiralling and circular patterns). Imagine that the (unseen) top of the figure is the top of the uterus, the fundus. The lines will be as dense here as they are at the lower end which represents the closed cervix. There is a slightly thicker layer of muscle at the top of the uterus (0.5-0.69 cm) than the lower end (0.4-0.45 cm). The network of elastic muscle illustrated here is sufficient to visualise how the fetus is contained within his incubator during pregnancy. Whenever he moves, he gets folded back into the fetal position.

The bottom of the figure is the cervix, tightly shut here. The longitudinal lines up to the first few rings surrounding the centre point in this illustration are not very elastic, they are high in collagen and low on muscle. This represents the closed system of pregnancy. (Even if the cervix is slightly open, as it can be towards the end of pregnancy, as long as there is more collagen than muscle at the lower end the uterus will still not open.)

Now imagine that there is a fetus presenting head first inside. Consider the effects of gravity alone if there was a hole at the lower end. Even without the effects of oxytocin, birth becomes inevitable once the collagen knot has been untied. Elastic stretch alone will force the balloon to expel its contents. Once contractions start to propagate they will spread along the lines of the network above. The direction of propagation depends on the alignment of the particular muscle cells that are stretched. In a trampoline the propagation is restricted to the length of stretched elastic but in the uterus, once it has been primed for labour, electrical signals from the stretched portion will propagate *further along* into unstretched muscle. The electrical signals triggering contraction could travel right up from the cervix to the fundus. The fundus will contract down forcibly because it has more muscle to contract and because of the laws of the mechanics of such shapes – a longer radius of curvature produces a bigger force (Haughton 1886). The circular muscle can only work by trying to fold the baby into a cylindrical shape, which will tend to steer him forwards towards the midline of the axis of symmetry, and eventually push him through it. As he passes through the cervix (or possibly before as well) the nerves of the vagina are stretched, which sends a signal to the pituitary to release large amounts of oxytocin to drive the second stage of labour.

Figure 34 is an approximation of the inside of the balloon that is the uterus before the onset of labour. Imagine the fetus inside heading towards the centre. If the collagen matrix surrounding the cervical muscle has now been broken down, it is inevitable that the uterus will open. The uterus is a balloon made up of muscle which contracts as a response to being stretched. The cervix can now be stretched, the baby's head has to stretch it and it has to open more.

I believe that this picture fits most of what we know about what the uterus does in labour and what happens to women in labour at home and in hospital. It can explain 'good' labour and 'bad' labour – the difference between coordinated and

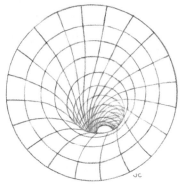

Figure 34: The baby's way out.

uncoordinated contractions. Positioning contractions happen in the latent stage of labour, before the cervix has started to open. If the woman stays at home and can move about as much as she wants, the baby will have the chance to position himself in the best way for leaving the uterus, but if she goes to hospital too soon and ends up staying on a bed, expecting labour to be painful, not realising that the pain is a signal to find a more comfortable position, she will not 'go with her body' and labour will become painful.

Any solid object outside the uterus may prevent the uterus being stretched and thus prevent positioning contractions taking place. This may lead to obstructed labour and even uterine rupture. Solid objects could include maternal body parts such as the spine or the brim of the pelvis, or external objects, usually the bed and possibly even monitoring belts. If contractions are unable to do their work in moving the baby, repeated attempts may lead to uterine exhaustion and prolonged labour.

The account above can explain why labour in an upright position is more efficient and less painful than labour in the supine position. The uterus needs to be free to be stretched so that it can respond by contracting. A certain amount of discomfort may be inevitable; the stretched muscle at the cervix will 'protest' at being unable to respond to stretch by contracting.

In this book I have been attempting to discover how the uterus works in normal labour. I feel that it would be helpful for the clinical community to revisit abnormal labour in the light of the hypotheses presented in this chapter. It might explain how dysfunctional labours could be turned round, giving some women the possibility of having a normal birth instead of needing a caesarean section. Certainly some midwives are already sceptical about the accepted accounts of uterine function. I will end this chapter with a quote to illustrate the point:

Contractions are measured according to how often they occur in a 10 minute period and are recorded as 2:10, 3:10, 4:10 etc.

To be considered 'effective' contractions need to occur 3:10 or more and last for 45 seconds or more. From a mechanistic perspective it would be impossible to progress through labour with 2 contractions or less every 10mins. I actually believed this for some time (again sorry to those women)...

What I now know is that a woman's contraction pattern is unique. I have witnessed women birth babies perfectly well with very 'ineffective' contraction patterns. The recent ones that stand out in my mind are: A woman with an occiput posterior baby whose contractions never got closer than 5 minutes apart and were mostly 7-10 minutes apart. And a first time mother who birth[ed] her baby with mostly 10 minute spaces between contractions. When left to birth physiologically women's labour patterns are as unique as they are. Unfortunately many midwives are unable to witness a variety of contraction patterns because individuality is not tolerated in the hospital setting. (Rachel Reed, www.midwifethinking)

7 The unique human pelvis

This chapter deals with the bony anatomy that nature has bequeathed to us via evolution, the survival and reproduction of the fittest. You can skip some of this chapter if you're not interested in how we acquired our brains, our culture, our unique mode of life and our oddly shaped pelvis, but I consider it part of the history of birth and I have to admit that human birth is much more problematic than birth in other mammals and want to know why. All other mammals give birth to young with small heads relative to their mother's pelvis and have a direct route to the outside world. We don't. Most of the blame can be put on the human pelvis which acquired a bend on the journey from ape to human. The line of hominids (prehumans) that led to us evolved into a creature with a large head to accommodate an expanded brain which had to twist and turn its way through a redesigned pelvis to be born. As the baby negotiated his way through the pelvis the mother tilted and rocked her pelvis to accommodate him but of course maternal behaviour left no traces in the fossil record.

There were many species of hominids, so the problem of a changed birth canal seems to have been solved more than once but hominids were stuck with relatively small brains for millions of years. Only one species lived to write the tale of its own history using its large brain (although the Neanderthals also managed to increase their brain power). Some must have fallen by the wayside but our own species evolved from the line that managed to find a way through this bottleneck.

The story of human evolution written into the fossil record is mostly the story of our bones. Features of the head and pelvis are so unique to the apes that started to walk upright, the hominids, that when such a fossil is unearthed, it is immediately apparent that it belonged to one of the hominid species. Humans are the only living descendants of one of those species.

We have inherited a large head which has to go through a pelvis which evolved to allow its owner to walk and run leaving both hands free to hunt or to gather – and to hold the baby. As soon as we started to diverge from our ape ancestors there had to be co-evolution of the maternal pelvis and the fetal head, both changing to accommodate each other for birth. The change to upright walking appears to have occurred first but could have continued only if infants survived to reproduce themselves. Then the baby's head got bigger and bigger to accommodate all that burgeoning brain power on the way to becoming fully human; brain size doubled and then doubled again. The jaw receded (man is the baby-faced ape – human faces are more like the faces of baby apes) and this, combined with the larger brain, made the skull more spherical.

At a conservative estimate of four generations per century, nature had at least 2,500 generations to select the 'right genes' to make the baby's head the right size to negotiate the mother's pelvis but some babies just don't seem to be able to fit. You will recall the evolutionary obstetric dilemma from Chapter One. The human pelvis became contorted. The hip bones were foreshortened and rotated upwards (see Figure 40, page 137), and the legs swung round to the sides. Birth became potentially problematic, particularly for babies presenting in the breech position (bottom first). The sad photograph of the bones of a mother and baby buried together with the fetal head still inside the mother's pelvis highlighted the obstetric dilemma, which is that women give birth to large-headed babies which only just fit through the pelvis. We can all be grateful that modern surgery has the means to rescue nature's mistakes.

How did we acquire a large head and oddly shaped pelvis?

Our human skeleton evolved from that of a primate who spent her life living in the trees, using all four limbs to clamber about in the forest canopy, distributing her body weight equally among four limbs. In the mid-nineteenth century, primates were known as quadrumana – four-handed rather than four-footed creatures. Primates used their fore and hind limbs for hanging on to branches, reaching for fruit, building their sleeping nests, and snatching their young out of harm's way. Other mammals evolved for other specialised ways of life. Bats learned to fly and used sonar to locate their food and navigate, lions learned to run for their dinner, and gazelles to run for their lives. Primates kept a more generalised body plan and continued to live in the forest, the habitat where mammals had originally evolved (towards the end of the age of dinosaurs) – but went up into the branches away from the dangers of the forest floor. Life in the treetops made it difficult to watch out for more than one offspring at a time – as family size decreased, brain size increased.

Why we came down from the trees, becoming two footed and two handed, no one really knows, but I subscribe to the aquatic ape hypothesis which postulates that upright walking, loss of fur, an aquiline nose and weeping salt tears came about through necessity when our habitat flooded and we became cut off from the African mainland. According to Elaine Morgan in *The Descent of Woman* and *The Scars of Evolution,* the ape who survived to become our ancestor learned to wade upright, then swim, it evolved an aquiline nose and subsisted on shellfish. Michael Crawford in the *The Driving Force* is also convinced by the aquatic ape hypothesis, considering marine food to be an excellent, easily foraged source of the essential fatty acids which are needed to make an 'expensive to maintain' brain. If you have ever wondered why a woman would ever choose to give birth in water – at first glance rather an extreme environment for such an activity – it may well be a trace memory of those long-distant times. I would even go so far as to say that without a method of birth where the weight of a mother's body was supported freely by water, the evolutionary changes to the pelvis enabling upright posture might never have been possible at all. Most of us have 'forgotten' that we evolved to give birth in water, but even after we decided we'd had enough of the seaside and returned to live on the land (climatic change seems the most likely explanation), we still managed to colonise every corner of the world. When forced to return to life on land, birth was still possible or we wouldn't be here. Perhaps we carried on giving birth in water for a time? While risk of hyperthermia seems an obvious drawback, doctors who care for sick newborn babies now give cooling therapy to babies thought to be at risk of brain damage after suspected oxygen deprivation during birth.

Natural selection took a few short cuts. Perhaps the most significant for our future development as humans was bringing forward the moment of birth to a time when the bones of the fetal skull had not yet fused into a solid skull and the plates of the skull could move to mould the head for birth. This effectively meant giving birth to a 'premature' baby which was more helpless than the offspring of other primates and would need more care from its mother – thus we can add co-evolution of maternal behaviour into the mix. The mother had to breastfeed for longer and to give more hands-on care if she wanted her offspring to survive. An extended childhood meant less need for behaviour hard-wired into the brain and gave more time for learning by experience. (Is this what kick-started mankind's cultural revolution?) There are still many unanswered riddles of evolution which could be solved by paying more attention to the mechanisms and process of birth and parenting.

Changes to the spine

Our body plan changed enormously to enable us to become habitual upright walkers balancing on two legs. Other primates have a 'C' shaped spine; offspring merely have to follow the pathway of the spine to be born through a narrow pelvic ring. In contrast, the human spine has four curves. The forward bend at the neck, the cervical spine, helps to balance the head, the thoracic curve compensates, the lumbar curve brings the spine towards the centre again and the sacrum and coccyx become anchoring points for structures which stop our abdominal and pelvic organs succumbing to the effects of gravity. Choosing to walk with our heads held high shifted the centre of gravity upwards. Without the lumbar curve, the vertebral column would lean forward, tipping us over, and without the backward bend it would be difficult to balance the head. Between them, the lumbar and thoracic curves direct the body's centre of gravity over the feet. The lowest sections of the spine are part of the pelvis itself. The sacrum, five fused vertebrae, forms the back of the pelvis, and the coccyx, the tailbone, hinges onto the sacrum. I used to wonder why we had a coccyx at all if we didn't have a tail to wag; wasn't it just a bit of extra weight to carry around with us, and why put something else in the way of the baby on his way out? However, delving into pelvic anatomy more deeply, I discovered that it provides attachment points for the ligaments and muscles of the pelvic floor which has rather a job on its hands – it has to contain and support the variable contents of pelvic organs like the bowel, the bladder and the uterus. I was similarly perplexed by the ischial spines which jut out into the pelvis at its lower end and look as if they'd also make the birth canal more difficult to navigate. They perform a similar function, providing anchoring points for ligaments to suspend the outlets of abdominal organs, such as the cervix of the uterus above the gaping empty space of the pelvic outlet.

The sacrum – the keystone

The human sacrum is the keystone of the pelvis. It connects to one moveable hip bone on each side – if our sacrum was fixed we wouldn't be able to walk. The three bones of the pelvis are joined together at the back by ligaments criss-crossing over the whole surface. The hip bones sweep round to meet at the front at the symphysis pubis. The pelvis is held together at the inside by ligaments and muscles that look like patterns created by a

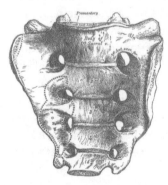

Figure 35: The 'sacred' sacrum.

child's toy, a Spirograph.

The evolution of the sacrum put an obstacle in the way of the emerging baby; the top of the lower bend of the 'S', the sacral promontory, marks the beginning of the birth canal. Now it became much more difficult to follow the usual mammalian birth plan for the offspring – follow the mother's spine to find the way out. It put an angle into the spine. Angles always imply a change of direction and if human babies had to be born facing a different direction, what better landmark could there be for the baby than a sacrum with a sharp angle at the top? The sacrum also curves in on itself and positively invites the baby's head to come in – and as we shall see – at a particular orientation.

Not only is the sacrum the keystone of the pelvis, it is a keystone for birth. It shows the baby the best way to enter the pelvis.

The name 'sacrum' is derived from the same Latin word as sacred – the ancients regarded the sacrum as holy. (I'm starting to agree with them.) It was believed that the sacrum could not be destroyed and that it was the part of the body that would allow someone to rise from the dead. This seems an odd notion for the western world which tends to believe that our humanity lies in our brains or perhaps our heart, but during birth *the sacrum moves outwards*. If movement of the sacrum is associated with birth, perhaps it is not so surprising that it should be associated with rebirth as well. In the days before patriarchal religion – when women were honoured for their role in bringing life into the world, when birth was deemed a sacred mystery, and when women chose their own positions for birth – they were attended by women who saw the sacrum move just before the birth. Birth was quite obviously a sacred event for all concerned. Now that birth mostly takes place in large hospitals we have lost the sense of the sacred. Besides, having put women upon their backs for birth, men could no longer see the sacrum move – indeed that position prevents it from moving – hence western women's problems in giving birth.

The curve of the cervical spine also has a role to play for birth, this time not for the mother but for her baby. We have far more movement at the neck than other mammals, we can bend our neck back 45 degrees and babies can move their heads back even more – indeed they have to be able to do this to negotiate the birth canal.

Changes to the pelvis

Not only is the sacrum a keystone, but the pelvis itself is also shaped like a keystone. Upright walking became possible only because the human pelvis adopted a crucial new role. The pelvis underwent a huge change of form and function in the journey from a body supported on all four limbs to upright walking as a hominid, while at the same time continuing to allow a safe passage through it for the next generation. In quadrupeds the pelvis needs to support only half the body weight, sharing that function with the shoulders and another two legs. In bipeds the pelvis had to support the weight of the whole body, head and all, while enabling the legs with their lockable knees to balance all that weight on the two small platforms of the feet.

The baby chimpanzee, with its small head, passes through a short straight tunnel on the way out. His small head can fit in virtually any direction and the rest of his body follows easily. The human baby, with a larger head, has to navigate a tunnel with a bend in it.

The hip bones turned inwards and the human pelvis acquired a bend at the front to turn it from a straight tube into a container. The pubic bones rotated upwards to become the lower front of the

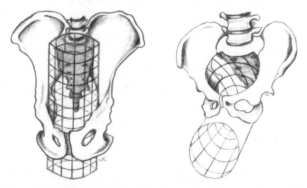

Figure 36: Small-headed chimps are born through a straight tunnel. Large-headed human babies are born through a tunnel with a 120° curve.

pelvic basin (half base, half front wall) and to provide anchoring points for the ligaments and muscles of a pelvic floor that now needed to support all the internal organs (in quadrupeds these merely needed to be suspended beneath the spine.)

Despite the fact that only humans need quite so robust a container to support their pelvic contents, the pelvis is named after the Latin word for basin. The pelvis supports the weight of the contents of the body at three levels. The uppermost space is above the sacral promontory and ends at those 'childbearing hips', the iliac crests. These are the widest part of the pelvis seen from the outside but do not pose a problem for birth; indeed they are useful for carrying toddlers on afterwards. This top level of the pelvis supports the weight of the organs above it. The lower end of this space is known as the 'obstetric inlet'. This is usually pictured from above so that the angle of entry of the fetal head (the drive angle) is lost. The sideways view shows the depth of that angle. This space extends from the obstetric inlet to the level of the ischial spines.

The next space is between the obstetric inlet and the ischial spines. The uterus has its own support system which suspends the cervix at the middle of the true pelvis, at an angle and above the level of the pelvic floor. Were it not supported separately, the weight of the pregnant uterus would compress everything beneath it. The points of attachment are the sacrum, the symphysis pubis and the ischial spines. The ischial spines are much more prominent in humans because they have more work to do. The cervix lies more or less behind the symphysis pubis.

When the cervix has dilated fully the head will move down to fill this space completely. The ischial spines are another landmark for the baby. They steer him towards the back of the pelvis to give him as large as possible a space to negotiate the notorious bend. The ischial spines are also used as landmarks by midwives and obstetricians to gauge how far the baby has descended.

The lowest level, the pelvic floor, supports the weight of the bladder and bowel on muscles that form a hammock running from front to back from the pubis at the front to the coccyx at the back. The hammock has a V-shaped gap at the front through which the baby will pass.

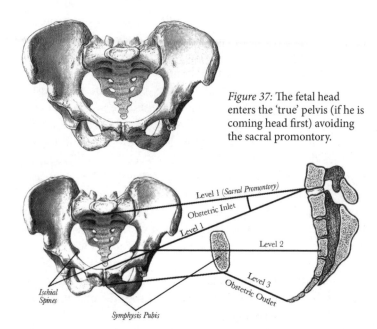

Figure 37: The fetal head enters the 'true' pelvis (if he is coming head first) avoiding the sacral promontory.

Figure 38: The three levels of the pelvis: level 1, the 'obstetric inlet', level 2, ischial spines, level 3 obstetric outlet (not to scale).

It might be easier for all if the tube had a nice circular cross-section all the way down but it doesn't. Not only does the tube have a bend but it is not even circular but oval, and moreover the orientation of that oval rotates 90 degrees after the bend in the birth canal.

We tend to think of this as a problem for birth but in fact the shape of the tube through the pelvis provides the baby with very clear signals about which way he is supposed to go. Visualised in its most simple form, the two largest sections of the baby's body, the head and the shoulders, are also ovals. The head is longest from front to back and the shoulders are widest from side to side. The baby has to twist and turn his way through a bent oval tube that has a different diameter at the inlet at the top from the diameter at the outlet. The next chapter will outline how he manages it.

8 Travelling through the pelvis

It has often appeared to me, as I sat watching a tedious labor case, how unnatural was the ordinary obstetric position for the parturient woman; the child is forced, I may say, upwards through the pelvic canal in the face of gravity, which acts in the intervals between the pains, and permits the presenting part of the child to sink back again, down the inclined canal. If we look upon the structure of the pelvis, more especially the direction of the pelvic canal and its axis, if we take into consideration the assistance which may be rendered by gravity, and, above all, by the abdominal muscles, the present obstetric position seems indeed a peculiar one. ... above all it is dictated by modern laws of obstetrics, the justice of which I have never dared question; we have all been taught their correctness, and we all thoughtlessly follow their dictates. There is no reason for assuming this position, though we are taught it; it is not reason, or obstetric science, but obstetric fashion which guides us, – guides us through our patients, and blindly do we, like all fashion's votaries, follow in the wake. (Dr G J Engelmann, *Labor among Primitive Peoples*, 1883)

One hundred and thirty years on obstetric opinion still prevails and now nearly all women give birth under obstetric care in hospital, on their backs, trying to give birth against the force of gravity. At the end of the chapter before last on how the uterus works in labour, the cervix has opened to its fullest extent, the uterus itself has become continuous with the birth canal and the baby has already started to move downwards through the pelvis. It's time to consider how the baby finds a pathway through his mother's awkward pelvis.

Childbirth, at the simplest level, requires a mechanism for getting one set of bones through another set of bones. For me, trying to piece together the mechanism of labour has been like

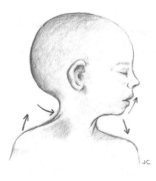

Figure 39: The baby can tilt his head up and down, rotate it, and hunch his shoulders to change his shape to fit through the birth canal.

trying to solve one of those seemingly intractable metal puzzles sometimes found in Christmas crackers. You twist and turn each piece against each other in turn until you find a way to slide them apart; you have to learn the trick of how to unlock them (and it's not a question of life or death for the metal puzzle!). The trick of human childbirth has much in common with the metal puzzle, moving two sets of bones around and against each other by trial and error. However, neither the mother nor her baby is made of metal. Although bones are relatively solid, the baby has a head that can mould where the skull plates have not yet joined and his head is attached to the rest of him via a partially rotating hinge at his neck; his shoulders can move up and down, reducing the width. The pelvis also has hinges.

Small movements of the pelvis

The mother's pelvis is not, after all, a rigid basin but has four joints with a surprising amount of movement in them. Mayes' *Textbook of Obstetrics* (1950) has a paragraph entitled 'The Dynamic Pelvis' which says, 'The study of the pelvis … is made on the "dead" pelvis of the dissecting room. It must be realised, however, that in Obstetrics we are dealing with a "living" pelvis, i.e. one in which there is movement.' There are small hinges on all four sides of the sacrum and, at the front of the pelvis, the symphysis pubis has some movement.

Figure 40 shows the iliac joints moving apart, they also seem to be able to move outwards increasing the outlet by as much as 2 cm (Russell, 1969). At the sacrum the bones are held

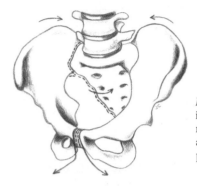

Figure 40: Space in the pelvis can increase by up to 30% through movement of the sacroiliac joints at the rear and at the symphysis pubis in front.

together by ligaments, a criss-crossing of ligaments at the back on the outside and connecting each side to the hip bones on the inside. The two front parts of the hip bones, the symphysis pubis, are able to move only a few millimetres, although more in pregnancy and labour (4-9 mm), and are joined by less mobile fibrocartilage. The hip bones are designed to move and, what is more, they have a greater range of movement in pregnant and labouring women. The amount of space in the pelvis can be increased by as much as 28% in the squatting position if the joints are free to move (Russell, 1969 cited in Polden and Mantle, 1990). The birth chairs of the 1970s and 1980s were designed with this increase in mind, for the benefit of western women who were unable to maintain a full squat for birth.

Opening the back

Sheila Kitzinger relates how Jamaican midwives talk about the mother not being able to give birth until she had 'opened her back' (Kitzinger 1993). 'Opening the back' destabilises the pelvis – the legs can no longer support the weight of the body. For the moment of birth itself we need to become quadrupeds again for a little while – we need the weight of our body to be supported by something other than just our legs.

'Opening the back' seems to correspond to upward movement of the rhombus of Michaelis, the kite-shaped area in the lower back that includes the three lower lumbar vertebrae and the sacrum. The shape of the rhombus of Michaelis implies that what the Jamaican midwives were seeing was

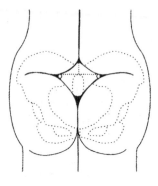

Figure 41: The evolved birth mechanism: the mother 'opens her back' at the rhombus of Michaelis.

the movement of the lumbar aponeurosis, a sheet-like area of tendon connected to the muscles it moves. Tendons relax during pregnancy, allowing more movement, thus the hips are able to dislocate. Jean Sutton (1996), a New Zealand midwife, was responsible for bringing knowledge of this movement at the pelvis back into midwifery thinking, and her work was written up by Sara Wickham in *The Practising Midwife* (2002). Sutton (quoted by Wickham) says: 'This wedge-shaped area moves backwards during the second stage of labour and, as it moves back, it pushes the wings of the ilea out, increasing the diameter of the pelvis.' The mid-pelvic cavity funnels in slightly; Mayes writes that the top of the inlet is 12.5 cm but only 10 cm at the bottom. Moving the sacrum out of the way increases the available space.

Sara Wickham related how she had seen women's backs move just before giving birth and assumed it was caused by the pressure of the head on the sacrum but Jean Sutton believes that it is caused by a nervous reflex, saying that, 'there must be some seriously large nerve plexus that triggers it off'. She has proposed that this could be linked with the Ferguson reflex, or that the plexus might be the G-spot, identifying parallels between the actions of women during orgasm and the second stage of labour (Wickham, 2002). The newly discovered internal body of the clitoris (see page 119 fits this description to the letter, the G spot is the location of the internal body of the clitoris. If this is the case, the vaginal contractions found at orgasm may have a role to play in birth. Women occasionally experience ejaculation at orgasm which implies that vaginal contractions involve a downward movement which could be evoked at birth. There certainly are some women who experience birth as orgasmic. Physiological links between the two processes seem likely given the release of large amounts of oxytocin both at orgasm and in birth.

Sara Wickham quotes Jean Sutton:

> When women are leaning forward, upright, or on their hands and knees, you will see a lump appear on their back, at and below waist level. It's much higher up than you might think; you don't look for it near her buttocks, you look for it near her waist. You can also feel it on the woman's back, it's a curved area of tissue that moves up into your hand, or you may suddenly see the mother grasp both sides of the back of her pelvis as the ilea are pushed out and she is suddenly aware of those muscles that have never been stretched before. Normally, the rhombus is only out for a matter of minutes, it comes out just as second stage starts, and it's gone back in again by the time that the baby's feet are born, in fact sometimes more quickly than that.

Groping towards an understanding of the reflex that Jean Sutton infers, I'm thinking it will be linked to the nervous reflex mechanism in female mammals which is linked to being sexually receptive. The lordosis reflex is seen in female mammals when they are hormonally prepared for sex (having high levels of oestrogen at mid cycle). Lordosis is elicited by a nervous reflex released by stroking the flanks (being mounted by a male) and by penetration, i.e. clitoral stimulation. In mammals this reflex moves the tail (coccyx) out of the way to allow penetration. Although humans have no tail, the same reflex would move the lower end of the sacrum outwards. This reflex could have been utilised by evolution to make more room for the passage of the baby in humans. Instead of being elicited by the action of the penis on the way in, it could be activated by the baby on the way out. The ventromedial nucleus of the hypothalamus, the area of the brain where the lordosis reflex can be elicited by electrical stimulation, is adjacent to the nervous input into the oxytocin-secreting part of the pituitary gland, and proximity suggests that the lordosis reflex may be linked to the oxytocin surge.

The nervous reflex that elicits lordosis in mammals also increases arousal, leading to increased adrenalin secretion. If this is what happens to initiate the movement of the sacrum, it happens just when mothers will need to be jerked back into a heightened awareness of the world and its dangers; when their baby is newly born and they are recovering from birth they will both be at their most vulnerable. If they are already in a place of safety will raised adrenalin, and high levels of oxytocin and endorphins, all be interpreted as a sense of being at one with the world?

Increased adrenalin secretion is associated with Michel Odent's fetal ejection reflex. He adopted the term 'fetus ejection reflex' to refer to 'the very last contractions before birth among humans, when the whole process has been undisturbed and unguided. This is a very short phase when, paradoxically, strong and effective contractions are associated with a rush of adrenalin so that the mother has a tendency to be alert when the baby is born'. (Odent, 1999) There is so much still to learn about neural mechanisms in birth. The link with lordosis is speculative but deserves further investigation.

Note that Odent refers to an undisturbed and unguided process. Sexual responses are notorious for being easily disturbed by environmental influences. Not only may the reflex be inhibited (by epidural anaesthesia which will quench nervous activity) but if the woman is on her back then the movement of the sacrum will be impossible. A side-lying or an all-fours position allows backwards movement of the sacrum but in the supine position there is nowhere for it to go. Modern obstetrics compensates for its disturbance of the natural process by infusing artificially high amounts of oxytocin. Artificial oxytocin promotes contractions but lacks any ability to influence the brain because it is infused from outside the brain and cannot cross the blood-brain barrier. When artificial oxytocin fails, then forceps or ventouse delivery is needed. Is it any wonder that there has been an increase in assisted deliveries? The profound lack of interest in the physiology of childbirth is one of the reasons for the high rates of intervention in modern childbirth.

Most women are unable to give birth using the fetus ejection reflex simply because the birth environment in obstetric units provides exactly the opposite of what is needed for women to access their innate powers. Critical elements of the birth process are disrupted. Obstetrics can only alleviate the situation of women who are deprived of the evolved reflex biomechanical process. Prevention is better than cure.

Large movements of the pelvis

What seems to be forgotten is that the mother can move her pelvis as a whole. She can rock from side to side, she can arch and hollow her back. She can tilt her pelvis by a fairly large angle forwards and backwards. She can tilt it from side to side by transferring weight from one knee to the other. She can rock her whole body forwards and backwards, she can lift one leg completely. These gross movements can enable her to move her pelvis *around* her baby giving him more space as he 'asks' for it. Reading clinical textbooks has made me realise that most doctors and midwives are taught the mechanics of childbirth as if there was only one position a pelvis could be in – attached to a passive patient flat on her back on a bed. Clinicians are taught to move the legs right back to put the mother in the McRoberts' position if the baby's shoulders get stuck, but that seems to be about the limit of the teaching about pelvic movement in standard clinical textbooks.

Once the baby has moved out of the uterus the mother can feel his head and shoulders directly and can make use of direct nervous signals to move. I'm not aware of any research relating to any of this, probably because women are usually put on their backs for birth, vastly reducing their available movement.

After the baby has entered the bony birth canal his movements seem to be dictated by the shape of his body, his neonatal (or rather fetal) reflexes, the shape of the tube and the barriers he comes up against. His mother is motivated by her need to relieve sensations of discomfort and pain and the desire to meet her child face to face as soon as possible. She can change the shape of the tube around him to accommodate his body.

Once her baby has moved out of the uterus and he is impinging on her vaginal walls, she can feel him directly. She knows she has reached the point of no return and absolutely must push him out now. She can feel him pressing on her rectum, and she knows what to do.

The first stage of labour has opened the cervix and started the baby off on his journey through that puzzling pelvis. The first part of his descent has taken place while he is still inside the uterus, the neck of the uterus being located within the pelvis. The pelvis has been engineered by evolution to guide a baby through, giving him the bony landmarks of the sacral promontory, the ischial spines and the symphysis pubis to fit his body into, through and under. The soft tissues of the pelvis also serve as guides, telling him where to aim and when to change direction. The mother can feel her soft tissues being stretched and can perhaps react subconsciously to what she feels. The positions the mother chooses to adopt make a huge difference as to whether she and her baby together manage to solve the head and pelvis puzzle. The mother needs to be able to move following her own instincts.

Birthing environment

Once again, the birthing environment, the people present and the furniture available, can encourage or discourage certain behaviours. Women need both physical and psychological support. What physical props are available to help the mother follow the urges of her body while she is pushing her baby out? Are there alternatives to the bed? Probably the attitude of the mother's caregivers has most influence on her behaviour. In hospital a few midwives prefer women to be in the lithotomy position, flat on the back, legs in stirrups. Mothers are instructed to 'Hold your breath and push' (the Valsalva technique, known as 'purple pushing' and which is not advisable because it decreases the oxygen supply to the baby). The latest Maternity Survey (2019) found that 24% of women giving birth under the category 'normal vaginal delivery' were delivered in the lithotomy position. I am shocked and appalled that this percentage has increased steadily year on year with each successive survey. This is what some midwives have been taught; this is how they are comfortable 'doing deliveries'. The increasing use of lithotomy position for normal birth might be linked to the increasing number of obstetric anal injuries (OASI, where the woman's rectum tears). One of the procedures in the 'care bundle' that has been developed to try and prevent these distressing injuries is an arguably brutal hands-on technique called the 'Finnish grip' designed to prevent the perineum from stretching just below the anus. It appals me. Correlation is not causation, but one could argue that OASI rates have increased in line with lithotomy rates. Spreading legs apart in the lithotomy position itself puts strain on the rectal area. Rather than advocate the Finnish grip, midwives could encourage women to give birth on all-fours or leaning forward so that the pressure of the fetal head is directed away from the rectum and towards the area designed to support it with blood filled shock absorbers – the clitoris. Obstetrician Gloria Esegbona is anxious to reduce the incidence of rectal tears and points out that moving the hip joints closer together also reduces tears. This may be why side lying is a better position than lithotomy – if the woman must be 'delivered' on a bed, she will at least be lying on one hip and gravity will use the weight of the other will bring it downwards.

Obstetric anal injuries are very rare in midwife-led environments where birth in lithotomy is rare. At the other end of the spectrum are midwives who move the furniture around and make sure that women have a full range of options available so women can get comfortable in whatever position they care to adopt, and say 'Push when you feel ready'. (To be fair, midwives have a lot of twisting, lifting and bending to do in their working lives and are prone to back problems. Some might suffer physical discomfort in delivering women in unusual positions.)

Water birth

There is one place in hospital where some lucky women are free to move the bones of their pelvis around for birth – in the birth pool. There are numerous videos of water births on YouTube and watching a few of these should be enough to make anyone realise the myriad of movements women can and do make to help their baby into the world. The buoyancy provided by water in supporting the mother's weight gives her a freedom of movement she could never have on dry land. However, water birth is still seen as outside the mainstream and although all midwives are supposed to be able to care for women choosing to labour in water, there are many ways of withholding that choice in an environment that is controlled by the caregiver. If there is only one room with a pool in it for every ten delivery rooms it is all too easy to say that the room is already in use. Even though we might have evolved to give birth in water, as proposed in the *Aquatic Ape Hypothesis* (Morgan, 1997), we've managed to give birth without its help for thousands of years and water birth is seen as 'alternative'.

The advantage of water is not only its buoyancy and the relief of pain but also in the sense of space and freedom. There are soft walls of the pool to lean against; in the pool, women can find so many different angles that wouldn't be comfortable or even possible on land. Position is as important in the second stage of labour as it is in the first stage because it enables a woman and her baby to work together to find the best angles.

Angles of birth

To return to dry land and the metal puzzle problem. Often the solution involves putting one piece against another at a specific angle. Get the angle right and the pieces almost fall apart from each other. The birth canal has an angle in it, the baby needs to enter facing one way and then change direction; directions imply angles of movement. Get the angles right and the baby can take the smoothest possible path through his mother's pelvis, get them wrong and he can get stuck. His position and thus his angle of entry are probably the most important factors in helping him to make a smooth exit. Movement of the pelvic joints, allowing the bony tube to expand while he is passing through, comes a close second. To manoeuvre through the pelvis and to exit the birth canal the baby makes good use of the largest angles that he can change – the angle of his head on his neck, nodding forwards (termed flexion) and tipping backwards (termed extension) and turning from side to side (rotation). These angles are determined by the range of movement at the baby's neck.

Working with or against all these angles in the mother's and baby's bodies is one direction that no one can change – gravity. It seems to me that the angle that is most disrupted by the supine position is the angle of the uterus to the first direction of travel through the pelvis. Contractions lift the uterus upwards and outwards – external toco transducers measure nothing more than the strain this movement puts on the maternal abdomen. In the supine position such contractions will need to work directly *against* gravity. Given that the pressure of the uterus lying on the blood vessels supplying it reduces blood supply and therefore deprives mother and baby of oxygen, a supine position seems positively absurd. Supine lying is totally irrational. Moreover, starting continuous monitoring – if that involves the supine position – when concerns about fetal well being have been raised is tantamount to fetal abuse.

Nature did her best in choosing the angle of the uterus to the vagina when adapting our pelvic architecture for upright walking – the female pelvis is a compromise between walking upright, staying pregnant and giving birth. However, nature's plans are easily thwarted when women are placed on their backs and the uterus has to work against gravity. Many of the angles are difficult to visualise simply by looking at two-dimensional anatomical drawings. Most drawings omit any question of movement, there is not so much as an arrow, and positions are illustrated from different viewpoints. Most of them assume that the woman is flat on her back. There are front, side and lower views of the pelvis; descent is drawn straight down (as though most women were, in fact, allowed to give birth upright).

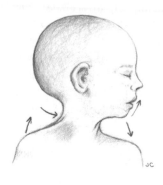

Figure 42: The baby can tilt his head up and down, rotate it, and hunch his shoulders to change his shape to fit through the birth canal.

The uterus is also drawn upright as if it were parallel to the mother's spine when it is, in fact, perpendicular to the pelvic brim. Pictures of the baby moving through the pelvis show him with his legs tucked up in the fetal position even after he has room to stretch his legs. Also, although his movements through the pelvis start while he is still inside the uterus, illustrations usually portray the uterus, cervix and vagina as continuous, with no indication of where they are in the pelvis. The pelvic floor muscles are never ever shown and yet they are thought to play an important part in guiding the baby round the curve of the pelvis. Using these diagrams it took me forever to get a picture into my head of how the baby might get down the pelvis to be born and a quick internet search showed that I'm not the only one to struggle.

It is significant that these illustrations give only the doctor's eye view of what is happening. If this is all the teaching material that is available for doctors and midwives, it's not really surprising that the vital importance of maternal position has been left out of the equation. I've been looking at things from the mother's and baby's eye view, a point of view which actually concerns what they can *feel* rather than what they can *see*. I also tend to visualise the mother upright, or even to turn her back into a quadruped and rotate her onto hands and knees. Trying to put it all into words has been a challenge, to say the least!

Eventually it dawned on me that even if we could visualise the 'anatomically correct' angles, the relationships between all these parts are not fixed. We can tilt our pelvis from side to side or from front to back; we can lift our legs up and out. We can even adopt the knee-chest position and take the pressure off the cervix altogether and allow gravity to help the baby manoeuvre himself into a better position. We can change the shape of our pelvis *around* the baby – if we have freedom of movement. We can even shift the baby around manually – the abdominal lift mentioned in Janie McCoy King's (1993) book *Back Labor No More* will be enabling the baby to move at the pelvic brim.

Drive angle

The near instantaneous release of stuck babies reported by Janie McCoy King may point to the importance of the drive angle in birth. First mentioned by E Gold (1950) in his paper entitled, 'Pelvic drive in obstetrics. An x-ray study of 100 cases', this is always mentioned as important when people are talking about position in labour. It is precisely this angle that is never accurately portrayed in the illustrations. The fetal head needs to be able to move down through the cervix at a perpendicular angle to the inlet of the pelvis before changing direction and travelling forwards. The position of the cervix is more or less fixed mid pelvis and becomes more fixed when the head has descended to fill it. Visualise the balloon again and it is apparent that the top of the uterus needs to be in a direct line with the cervix in order for contractions to have the best effect in opening it. For labour to proceed normally, the fetal head needs to be 'well applied' to the cervix. The outward movement of the uterus during contractions helps the head to find the optimal angle of entry. Until the cervix has effaced, the tunnel of the pelvis is not 'revealed' to the fetus. As the cervix opens the tunnel becomes apparent (this is what Milani-Comparetti meant by the 'invitation to softness') and the baby tips his head into it and travels on down. When a woman is in an upright posture and leans forward, gravity will help to optimise the angle.

Polden and Mantle (1990), obstetric physiotherapists, describe the drive angle this way:

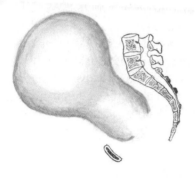

Figure 43: Concept of the drive angle. Lifting the abdomen may improve the drive angle.

… during contractions the shape of the abdomen alters, the fundus moves forward so that the long axis of the uterus and the thrust of the muscle are brought forward into the appropriate line and meet the cervix and the vagina at the best angle (drive angle) to propel the fetus into the vagina. This forward tilt (anteversion) occurs more easily if the woman is upright or lying on her side, for gravity opposes it in the supine position. It is of interest that women instinctively lean forward.

Possible mechanism

Sometimes the cervix will open fully before the baby descends at all. The abdominal lift may help the baby to find a tunnel ready and waiting for him, perhaps activating the Moro reflex whereby on tipping back the head by an inch, he tries to stretch his limbs (although he doesn't have room in the uterus to do this) then bring them back into the body. This mechanism would account for the very speedy births that can occur after an abdominal lift reported by McCoy King (1993), Simkin and Ancheta (2000) and Gail Tully of the Spinning Babies website (2014).

Cardinal movements

The movements of the baby through the pelvis are known as the cardinal movements. These have been the subject of much speculation for many years. Like contractions, the cardinal movements are rarely explained. They also 'just happen' although at least the baby is credited with being able to move – even if his mother is still lying passively! A good active early labour should put the baby fair and square into the most favourable position for a smooth passage through the pelvis. If a woman is on her side, or the first part of her labour has been rushed through with artificial oxytocin, or the uterine pain positioning signals have been filtered out with epidural anaesthesia, her uterus may not have been able to position him squarely; sometimes he can enter the pelvis with his head extended, or tipped slightly to one side, termed asynclitism. This will make his passage through the pelvis more difficult. However, let's assume that he is in a good position and, having got to this good position, the uterus has contracted around him to put him in the fetal position – which is of course the shape of the uterus itself – so he has a rounded back and head tucked in (flexed).

The cardinal movements are: 1) flexion, 2) descent, 3) engagement, 4) internal rotation, 5) extension, 6) restitution and 7) external rotation. These movements all refer to the position of the head. Far less attention is paid to the position of the shoulders and yet these are wider than the head. The baby can, however, reduce the width of his shoulders as he moves through the pelvis by hunching one up and the other down.

A nicely numbered list is easier to remember when it comes to exam time, but real life is not so neat and tidy. Descent must precede engagement and, of course, the baby must descend all the way through active labour. A well positioned baby is already flexed into the fetal position and engagement is a gradual process which has already involved 45 degrees of rotation. There seems to be some dispute about exactly where the baby is when internal rotation and extension happen and how and why these movements occur. Anne Frye (2004) refers to Borell and Fernström (1959) who x-rayed mothers in labour and found that in first-time mothers the head rotates above the curve of the birth canal while for mothers who have given birth before, rotation takes places lower down the birth canal. This difference between mothers who are giving birth for the first time and those who are repeating the event can be explained by the condition of the pelvic floor muscles. Rotation appears to take place at the pelvic floor and seems to depend on good muscle tone there; first-time mothers will have better muscle tone because their muscles have not been stretched before. Failure to rotate is a common problem when women have epidural anaesthesia and these muscles are lax.

Nearly all of these movements occur inside the mother's body and, apart from Borell and Fernström's x-rays and one short MRI scan of a mother who agreed to give birth to her baby in a scanner, none has been seen directly. Most of these movements have been worked out by feeling the position of the baby's head on vaginal examination at a particular place relative to the bones of the mother's pelvis, and most of the time the mother will have been in a supine position – if only because it is far easier to examine a woman vaginally when she is lying down.

The journey

The following account is how I visualise the journey of a well positioned baby through the pelvis. The baby fits the top of his head across the pelvic brim, then turns inwards 45 degrees to avoid his mother's sacral promontory. Contractions push him downwards and he carries on turning in towards his mother's back, following the inward curve of the saucer-shaped sacrum with his forehead. He tucks his chin to his chest as he does so. Now he is facing squarely into the curve of his mother's sacrum. The back of his head is following the shorter path of the symphysis pubis. His forehead leading the way, he follows the longer outside curve of the sacrum and coccyx to its end. When his forehead has moved past the end of the coccyx and the back of his head has cleared the bases of the pubic arch his head is free to 'untuck'; he extends it and his head is born. The back of his head is born first and his face is revealed from the top of his brow downwards as he continues to tip his head back (extension). But now his shoulders encounter the back of the pubic arch and stop further forward movement. His shoulders must now twist to follow his head. Uncomfortable with a twisted neck, he turns his head to one side and as he turns his head his shoulders can now follow and he can be born. The rest of him follows easily.

Another way of looking at it is to visualise him doing a third of a backward somersault (120 degrees) starting with an eighth turn to get his face past the sacral promontory, followed by another eighth turn so that the back of his head follows the internal contour of the symphysis pubis, while his forehead follows the curve of the sacrum.

These movements describe the pathway of a baby positioned in the ideal place for the journey. This is a mother's attempt to understand how babies get born. I don't propose trying to describe any other pathway but it's worth considering what might happen when the starting position is not ideal. This is why I so passionately believe that we have to change attitudes about mothers' positions in labour.

Other starting positions

When I had my first baby the 'cooperation card' (the notes I carried) with the usual medical hieroglyphics included a whole column of 'ROPs'. This told the professionals what position my baby was in relative to the pelvic inlet. Translated into medical English it meant 'Right Occiput Posterior' and translated into ordinary English this meant that the back of my baby's head (O for the baby's occiput) was at the back of my pelvis (P for my posterior) on my right hand side (R). This is not the best starting position for babies and usually leads to a very painful labour. I had no idea that this was the case until I read an article in *Midwifery Matters* entitled, 'Sorry, love, it's OP' (Jessop, 1989.) Apparently, everyone except for me and my husband knew that I was in for a hard time in labour. A baby facing outwards means that the hard part of the baby's head presses against the back of the mother's pelvis, causing near constant pain. This is known a 'back labour'. Looking back on it, I'm angry with the obstetrician who thought that it would be a good idea to start my labour off by breaking the waters – this is another way of making birth more painful than it need be and is known as a 'dry labour'. (The amniotic fluid evens out the pressure inside the uterus; once the waters are broken, the baby's movements become sharper leading to 'spikier' contractions.) As it turned out my labour was hard and fierce but the pain was bearable when I sat upright and only excruciating when I tried lying down.

I was just unlucky. After resting at the pelvic brim for some weeks, most babies enter their mother's pelvis upside down and sideways (LOT, ROT – T for transverse) then turn 45 degrees inwards to face her internal sacroiliac joint (LOA or ROA – A for Anterior) thus avoiding the sacral promontory, the baby's first landmark. For some reason (probably because I am a singer with strong abdominal muscles) my baby found it more comfortable to face outwards at the end of pregnancy and perhaps didn't have space to turn.

Whatever the position of the baby, as long as he is head down or head up and the presenting part will fit into the internal part of the pelvis, it is usually possible for him to be born vaginally so long as the mother is free to follow her instincts and move around and she manages to avoid obstetric intervention. Wendy Savage, an English obstetrician, quotes her Dutch colleague, Professor Kloosterman, who said:

> … we obstetricians will have to listen to the ever louder voices of the public and we must try to learn from the lesson of history, that is:
> 1. To accept that childbirth is more than a study object for obstetricians, it is every human being's concern.
> 2. To accept that thorough study of one aspect can make us blind for other aspects, sometimes even more important.
> 3. To accept that the great and admirable improvement in obstetric care is only important in the handling of pathology. In no way can we improve a normal pregnancy and labour for a healthy woman; we can only change it but not for the better. (Savage, 1989)

It is midwives who can improve a normal pregnancy and labour by listening to women, supporting them in labour, encouraging them to believe and trust in the ability of their bodies to give birth, and by allowing mothers freedom of movement and freedom of position. Some midwives become dab hands at warding off unwanted and unwarranted obstetric attention, but it is becoming more and more difficult to do this as obstetric guidelines in hospital, and even at home, become ever more rigid.

Apart from explanations such as the baby rotating on the pelvic floor, according to the textbooks, the cardinal movements, like contractions, 'just happen' but I have tried to visualise why, where and when they happen. For example, why does the baby usually turn inwards? It might be caused by one of the neonatal reflexes. The rooting reflex is elicited by stroking the baby's cheek and makes him turn his head towards the cheek that is stroked. It is assumed that this reflex helps the baby find the mother's breast after birth, but if his cheek comes up against the sacral promontory as he comes down into the pelvis, it would also make him turn in towards the mother's back on entering the pelvis.

Reflex	Stimulus	Response	Use in labour
Stepping reflex	Held upright with feet touching the ground	Walking motions with legs and feet	Stimulating the fundus (the top of the uterus) to contract
Moro reflex	Allowing the head to fall back an inch	Arms and legs first extend then pull back towards the body	Getting into the pelvic inlet
Asymmetric tonic neck reflex	Turning the head to one side	As the head is turned, the arm and leg on the same side will extend, while the opposite limbs bend	Restitution (realigning head and shoulders after the birth of the head)
Tonic labyrinthine reflex	Lying on the back, tilting the head back	The back stiffens and can even arch backwards, the legs straighten, stiffen and push together, toes point, arms bend at the elbows and wrists, and the hands make fists	Extension of the head to get under the pubic arch. The pushing feet stimulate the fundus to contract
Galant reflex	Stroking along one side of the spine	Trunk and hips move toward the side of the stimulus	Rotation into the mother's sacrum
Rooting reflex	Stroking the baby's cheek	Turns head towards the stimulus	Rotation into the pelvic inlet

Table 2: The reflexes that are possibly involved in labour.

Even if I am wrong about how the fetal reflexes are involved in birth, it does look as if the shape of the pelvis and the shape of the baby's head are designed to fit together to go past each other during birth. Just as the metal puzzle pieces glide past each other to separate, so two bodies move past each other for a baby to be born. And it looks as though the 'ancients' were right in attributing magical powers to the sacrum, that saucer-shaped bone is the keystone. I cannot believe that we were meant to deny it half its powers by lying on top of it!

The baby will work out the best way to move through his mother – even if we don't understand it.

Rachel Reed, Midwifethinking.com

To conclude, I believe that in order to make full use of these movements, and to increase the available space, women can turn back into quadrupeds and support themselves using hands (or elbows) and knees. Having said that, it would be as wrong to dictate all-fours birth as it would be to dictate supine, semi-sitting or side-lying birth. Women's bodies will be able to tell them how best to move. During my son's birth my body had 'asked' me to lie on my side for the birth itself. Twenty years later I'm wondering whether this was because my pelvis was already destabilised by pressure from his head – to this day his head is asymmetric – perhaps birth on a birth stool or on all-fours would have dislocated my sacroiliac joint completely and, somehow, my body knew it. Luckily, I was in a place where I could hear my instincts and act on them.

To me, the usual Western birth position now seems positively barbaric. It makes absolutely no sense to immobilise women when they could be shifting their pelvis around to suit the needs of their baby. The mother's body can choose for itself the optimal position if she can only hear the signals it is giving. Perhaps one day someone will be able to describe the cardinal movements of the mother; or perhaps they won't. Perhaps every birth is different, and every woman chooses different movements to give birth to that particular baby.

I started this chapter with a quote from a doctor who believed 140 years ago that his colleagues were misguided. Engelmann pointed out that doctors were not inclined to spend time 'watching a tedious labor case'. Neither do doctors have the time today; they are called in only when needed, and most of the manoeuvres they are required to do are performed on a woman lying on her back on the bed, often with her legs in stirrups. Most doctors will never have seen a woman giving birth in any other position. They will never have seen a woman's back 'opening'.

Ina May Gaskin, an American midwife, talks of women having to find their 'inner monkey' when giving birth, 'Let your monkey do it!' she says. As we have seen from the above, monkeys should have an easy time of it from the bones' point of view. We may not be monkeys (we have no tails and we are more closely related to the apes, our closest relative is a chimpanzee) but we are still primates, who just happen to possess an altered pelvis which has been fine tuned by natural selection to allow us to give birth safely.

9 The hazards of technological birth

Most technology is designed to save time, labour, money or life. Obstetric technology can and sometimes does save lives, but for the most part it has been designed to save the doctor's time and the hospital's costs measured by the costs of providing a room for labour and a midwife to attend a woman. Fetal monitors are very expensive but are considered money well spent because they may save on the cost of a midwife's time – arguably a woman on a monitor can be left alone – and they may save money on the cost of litigation should there be an adverse outcome to the birth. I would argue that saving midwives' time is counterproductive. What women need most of all while giving birth is human support, and the time and attention of a midwife they have met before. They need a nest for labour in a relaxed environment with comfortable furniture, where they can be relieved of the pressures of the outside world. They need to be able to hear and listen to what their bodies are telling them and to have the opportunity to follow those instructions. This approach in itself shortens labour. Fetal monitors may actually prolong labour by keeping a woman on her back.

There is hardly a technology in the history of childbirth that has not constrained and limited a woman's ability to move freely and adopt positions of her own choosing. Technology in most cases is controlled by caregivers and thus puts limits on how much control a woman can have over the way her labour is managed. Such is the appeal of technology today that most people think that babies should be born in hospital where they have all the technology 'just in case', but technology proves itself a false god, usually causing more harm than good. While I certainly wouldn't like to return to the days when the only technology was hooks and crotchets to dismember and extract a dead fetus in the hopes of saving the life of the mother, the potentially life-saving technology of forceps was quickly turned into life-threatening technology.

Forceps

Barber surgeons were licensed to use surgical instruments and were called in by midwives to extract the fetal remains after a baby was thought to have died in labour, a truly dreadful job because the mother often died as well (this was before the day of the stethoscope which was not invented until 1816). A French barber surgeon, Peter Chamberlen, must have been delighted to invent an instrument, the obstetrical forceps, which was capable of delivering a live baby. Now the man-midwife could be called to a birth, but the Chamberlen family were to keep the invention a secret for 150 years. The sons migrated to England around 1600, bringing the forceps with them and describing themselves as man-midwives. The elder son was convincing enough to achieve the position of accoucheur at the royal court (until then midwives had been responsible for royal births) and his brother tried but failed to set up a midwifery society to gain control of birth through the midwifery profession. The scheme was vetoed by the Privy Council on the advice of the College of Physicians that midwives should continue to be licensed through the Church. Having failed to gain access to the midwifery profession, the next generation of Chamberlens trained as doctors and thus birth became a medical event, for the rich at least. The last Chamberlen died in 1728 and the family secret became common knowledge within ten years. The mere fact that forceps were kept a closely guarded secret kept in one family for so long shows the financial vested interest in birth. Rich families could afford the Chamberlens and their forceps; poor women continued to call the midwife.

It took 150 years of trial and error before the man-midwife with his forceps could be greeted with anything other than fear and trepidation. Although forceps have saved some babies' lives, there can be little doubt that they have destroyed countless others through over-zealous intervention caused by impatience on the part of doctors. Quite apart from the physical damage they did to the mother and her baby, before the advent of sterilisation techniques for surgical instruments, they were the means of introducing infection, which put the mother's life at risk. Furthermore, the mother had to be flat on her back and immobile and this changed the cultural expectation of the normal maternal position for labour and birth, at least in hospital. The mere existence of forceps created a problem for obstetrics to solve. Many more lives were lost in the early days of maternity hospitals where the doctors learnt their trade so that they could go on to earn fat fees from middle class mothers labouring at home in relative safety. And this is not just ancient history; in the USA in the 1930s virtually all babies born in hospital were delivered by forceps, the obstetricians routinely performed an episiotomy (cutting the perineum) and 'lift out' – it saved their time and earned them higher fees. Even today some babies die in botched forceps deliveries; practical skills still have to be learnt by experience. At the Birthrights conference, Dignity in Childbirth, in 2013 a mother related the death of her baby delivered by forceps wielded by an inexperienced doctor. Numerous studies have shown that women adopting an upright position for labour and birth are less likely to have a forceps delivery and therefore more likely to have a normal labour and birth.

Doctors wielding forceps never saw normal birth with a woman in any position other than supine and, since midwifery education was designed to train the type of birth attendants doctors wanted, essentially obstetric nurses, the question of birth position was not on the curriculum. Midwives training on an apprenticeship model, supporting women labouring at home, could learn the importance of position; their hospital-trained counterparts learned to label such positions 'alternative'.

Vacuum extraction

Ventouse is the French word for sink plunger, a household device used to unblock drains. It works by creating a vacuum. Calling vacuum delivery 'ventouse' sanitises the process by obscuring the reality of the method of extraction. There are advantages to vacuum delivery over forceps delivery. The suction cap can be introduced without cutting an episiotomy and some modern obstetricians will use it to ease the fetal head along, then release the suction and 'allow' the woman to complete the birth using 'maternal effort' (Gould 1998). Delivery by vacuum extraction owes its existence to the development of a device invented to treat the ill effects of delivery by forceps. The 'air tractor' was originally designed to treat depressed skull fractures, a condition caused by pressing the blades of the forceps too closely together. Its application in obstetrics was described by Neil Arnott, a Scottish obstetrician, in 1829:

> We have spoken ... under the name of pneumatic tractor, of a circular piece of leather, or similar soft substance, kept extended by included solid rings or radii, as being adapted to some purposes of surgery. Now it seems peculiarly adapted to the purpose of obstetric surgery, viz, as a substitute for the steel forceps, in the hands of men who are deficient in manual dexterity, whether from inexperience or natural inaptitude.
>
> With it the physician can dispense with anaesthetics and reduce the expulsive stage of labour to a few minutes, instead of hours. The agony of child-birth will be reduced to an infinitesimal degree without incurring any risk or inflicting any injury on either the mother or the child, and many lives will be saved which would otherwise be lost. [The author had] ... used the Tractor in five cases and in each case effected delivery with it in five minutes ... an instrument capable of producing such beneficial results is certain to be universally employed within a comparatively brief period. (Quoted in Baskett, 2009.)

The claim that it would reduce the agony of childbirth *to* an infinitesimal degree is grossly exaggerated. It might be nearer the mark to say that pain would be reduced *by* an infinitesimal degree. Again, the circular piece of leather introduces a source of infection into the birth canal and again it saves the doctor's valuable time. (He is not paid by the hour but by the number of cases he treats.)

The invention of the vacuum extraction apparatus may

have alleviated obstetric problems during the birth itself, but the fundamental problems solved by assisted delivery, malposition and prolonged second stage, were likely to be the end result of restriction of maternal movement earlier in labour. Even if forceps and ventouse aren't used, the damage done to mothers and babies by changing the default position for labour and birth to horizontal is incalculable and continues today. A 2010 survey by the Care Quality Commission found a rate of 16% of unassisted vaginal deliveries in the lithotomy position in England – a country where midwifery care is the norm. In 2019 this rate had increased to 24%. The problem is getting worse, not better. In some places midwives are allowed to perform ventouse deliveries. I am not alone in having mixed feelings about this; midwife ventouse practitioners themselves write of the temptation to intervene inappropriately (Charles, 1999), but keeping obstetricians away from women minimises disempowerment of the labouring woman.

A student midwife writes:

> To me, the difference between a midwife I'd never met coming in to do the lift out and a doctor coming in … wouldn't be much. The only reason I'd feel the benefit of continuity is if it was the midwife caring for me that would be doing the lift out. This isn't an area of career development I plan to pursue. I feel it is running into the realms of medical practice which isn't something I want to do.

Pain relief

When it was first introduced, there were theological qualms about using anaesthesia for labour – didn't God decree that women should suffer in labour? Queen Victoria's wholehearted endorsement of chloroform started to change the culture: '…I was taken ill early on the morning of the 7th & a boy was born to great happiness to me. Dr Snow administered "that blessed Chloroform" & the effect was soothing, quieting & delightful beyond measure…' James Simpson, a Scottish obstetrician, had discovered its anaesthetic properties in November 1847 and within days he was administering it to women in labour;

no clinical trials were needed then and there were no drug regulations to adhere to in those days. Once again a new technology had a detrimental effect on maternal positioning; an anaesthetised woman couldn't remain upright for labour and birth.

The introduction of nitrous oxide and air alleviated matters as far as analgesia was concerned. After clinical trials in hospital, the Minnitt apparatus was designed for use in the domestic setting. Since 1965 Entonox, a 50:50 mix of nitrous oxide and oxygen, has been used instead. It is still widely used in hospital birth and a woman's mobility depends only on the length of the pipe. The other virtue of Entonox is that it is controlled by the woman herself. She decides when she needs it and applies the mask and inhales accordingly.

The next on the hierarchy of pain relief is morphine in its various forms. Queen Victoria might also have used her era's universal panacea for pain, laudanum, a mixture of opium (from which morphine is extracted) and red wine, but since both alcohol and morphine inhibit uterine contractions her doctors might have thought better than recommend it. Opiates are still widely used, although today's preparations omit the alcohol. Many hospitals now prefer diamorphine (heroin) to pethidine but the relative risks and benefits are still disputed (Ullman *et al*, 2010). The inhibitory effect of opiates on contractions is glossed over in the medical literature. Since the body produces its own endorphins (known as the opiate within) during labour, doctors must think that prescribed opiates are innocuous. However, it is considered advisable to withhold opiates within two hours of the birth because they cause respiratory depression in the newborn – this is treated with naloxone, an opiate antagonist. I looked at the role of naturally secreted endorphins in labour in my last book (Jowitt, 1993) and concluded that their role is to regulate uterine activity according to the physical and emotional stress of the mother and to act as a physiological brake on the positive hormonal feedback mechanisms of labour. This view is still controversial although nothing I have seen since counteracts it and a possible mechanism has emerged, the inhibitory action of nitric oxide (not to be confused with nitrous oxide) on smooth muscle.

The scientific establishment has gone quiet on the subject of endorphins; I suspect that this is because they have been taken up by the alternative health movement, which has made them a less 'respectable' field of study. The natural childbirth movement remains convinced that you cannot have too much of a good thing – that the natural pain relief and euphoria associated with high levels of endorphins are good for women and their babies. This may be the case when a birth has gone well but, when birth has been traumatic, endorphins are still raised and there is dysphoria instead of euphoria. High levels of beta-endorphin are associated with post-traumatic stress disorder. Endorphins may act to heighten whatever mood one is experiencing. Whatever the final verdict on the role of natural endorphins in labour may be, manufactured opiates are labelled narcotics – sleep-inducing substances – and since the bed is the usual place for sleep, they are unlikely to be useful during active labour when the bodies of the mother and baby are working together to position the baby for birth. The late Mary Cronk, a midwife who started to practise before district midwifery was brought into the NHS, found that very small doses of pethidine (doses which some might consider 'homeopathic') could be useful, particularly for first-time mothers experiencing a long latent phase of labour. Pethidine is valuable for many women for its action as a muscle relaxant. She found that it enabled exhausted women to relax and sleep – the bed does have its uses in labour. However, she never used diamorphine, and never used pethidine in hefty doses (Cronk, 2014, personal communication).

Epidural

Continuous epidural anaesthesia was first tried in 1941 (Hingson, 1942). An early study of 300 women in 1943 showed that it disrupted the baby's movements leading to more occiput posterior ('face to pubes') labours, and while the anaesthesia abolished the pain of contractions, back pain persisted. More often than not babies failed to rotate and 70% of first-time mothers needed a rotational forceps delivery (Siever and Mousel, 1943). Rotational forceps are dangerous for the baby and today delivery is likely to be by caesarean section. Seventy years later, although the least harmful types of anaesthetic and the optimal doses are used, these drawbacks remain.

Blocking painful contractions means abolishing signals to the mother to move, making the uterus unable to position the baby for his journey through the pelvis. Women are more likely to need augmentation with artificial oxytocin because the nerves activated by the stretch of the cervix and upper vagina and signalling for oxytocin are blocked. Since they can no longer feel their stronger artificially induced contractions, they need electronic fetal monitoring.

Intravenous lines are set up for hydration because epidurals lower the blood pressure, thereby reducing oxygenation of the baby's blood. A catheter is inserted to drain urine because the woman loses the signal to urinate. Babies fail to rotate through the pelvis and need to be extracted by ventouse or forceps.

'Walking' epidurals are available but the increased movement does not seem to help women give birth without assistance. With an epidural there appears to be no clinical advantage in being upright for the birth (Kemp *et al*, 2013). Women who are most at risk of complications are given epidurals in case they need a caesarean and immobilised in bed so that their 'less productive' contractions which are not opening the cervix can be monitored. The drawbacks to epidurals go on and on.

Lack of access to epidural is cited as a drawback to birth outside hospital (although women can always transfer to obstetric units for pain relief if they need it). Epidural anaesthesia is recommended when labour requires augmentation by artificial oxytocin. There is a school of thought (seen in response to press articles about natural childbirth) that says that it is barbaric for women to give birth without an epidural. While some women wouldn't dream of labouring without an epidural, many much prefer to do without it if they possibly can. Epidurals disrupt the course of labour, thus increasing the need for instrumental deliveries. Epidurals are often given to relieve professional distress (Leap, 2000).

Measuring labour – birth by numbers

Length of labour

For the first few hundred years of medicalised childbirth, doctors were unable to do anything other than to break the waters to speed up labour. Until the invention of drugs to treat infection, the only other option, caesarean section, remained an intervention of last resort. Drugs used to speed up labour were still at the experimental stage. Doctors tended to limit their interventions to the second stage of labour, leaving midwives and nurses to manage the first stage. While birth still took place in the home and when pupil nurses and midwives provided much of the care during labour, women could labour in their own good time, making use of the comfortable furniture in their own homes – the sofa, kitchen worktops, the ironing board, the toilet – but then birth moved to the hospital and doctors were able to speed up labour with drugs and to deal with the consequences.

Now that the first stage of labour could be managed medically, as soon as women became under medical control the clock started ticking. Sheila Kitzinger has described the clock as an 'unevaluated technological intervention that has a major impact on the conduction of birth'.

Before doctors became interested in managing the early part of labour, degree of cervical dilatation was recorded in 'fingers', afterwards, dilatation was recorded more 'scientifically' in centimetres – but whatever the unit of measurement, both were still estimates.

However, numbers can be plotted on a graph. Friedman introduced the partogram in 1954 (Friedman, 1954). The partogram was a visual representation of the progress of labour which plotted time against degree of cervical dilatation in centimetres and included space for other aspects of labour that could be recorded numerically: number of contractions per ten minutes, fetal heart rate, descent of the fetal head in relation to the ischial spines, maternal pulse and temperature. One centimetre of dilatation per hour became the rule of thumb and it became axiomatic that contractions would increase in both strength and frequency. From then on the clock dominated the labour room. Women were 'allowed' so many hours to achieve full dilatation before action was taken for 'failure to progress'. Labour could now be managed scientifically.

In the 1950s the only action available was to break the waters but soon after came artificial oxytocin which was used liberally until some doctors noticed that it raised the rate of admission of babies to special care baby units. Obstetric care is not safe today unless it takes place where there are specialised baby units to rescue babies harmed by overenthusiastic obstetric intervention.

Measuring contractions

Tocodynamometry was first invented around 1870 as a research tool to look at the effect of various drugs, particularly anaesthetic agents and pain-relieving drugs, on contractions. A fluid-filled balloon catheter was inserted into the uterus through the cervix and linked directly to a recording device. Internal pressure monitoring is essentially the same today, although the balloon that measured pressure mechanically has been replaced by a catheter-tip pressure-transducer.

However, internal uterine pressure monitoring was invasive and inserting it risked breaking the membranes which protect the baby by spreading out the force of the contraction over the entire uterus. This led to attempts to measure contractions externally, from outside the body. At first this required the entire recording unit to be strapped to the mother's abdomen but in the 1930s a strain gauge attached to an abdominal belt was developed. In 1949 Samuel Reynolds published the second edition of his seminal work, *Physiology of the Uterus*. In it he introduced the notion that: 'Cervical dilatation in women is the result of a gradient of diminishing physiologic activity from the fundus to the lower uterine segment.' He had come to this conclusion by recording strain externally on the abdominal surface in nine different places, thinking that he was measuring the activity of the underlying uterus in nine different places. The synchronicity of the downward gradient looked compelling. It is Reynolds' work that is the basis for the notion that the contractions of active labour always follow this pattern, that contractions originate from the top of the uterus and spread downwards. He was measuring the effect of just one contraction on the shape of the abdominal wall in different places. The synchronicity and the downward gradient were an illusion.

Writing about the limitations of monitoring contractions externally, Nagel and Schaldach (1983) say:

> Despite very thorough investigation, agreement has still not been reached as to what, in fact, this transducer is measuring. The 'hardness' of the uterine wall is a complex parameter which depends upon the wall tension, radius, wall thickness, internal pressure, transverse elasticity and the hardness of the uterine musculature, and is just as involved in the measurement, as is the deformation of the uterus and its 'erection' during contractions. A further component of the measured signal results from the elastic nature of the transducer attachment. It can thus readily be appreciated that external tocography does not permit any statement about the absolute contraction amplitude nor the absolute level of the basal pressure or tone. All that we can obtain is an impression of the relative intensity of uterine contractions and changes in the basal pressure. Even this restricted performance may only be obtained when it is ensured that the transducer remains at its original site throughout the recording period and that the measuring conditions are not changed by any alteration of the patient's position. In very many cases these requirements cannot be met; indeed the maintenance of a given position by the patient might even be dangerous for her and her fetus.

Buhimschi *et al* (2003) also warn that:

> … the information obtained is limited, may not detect all uterine contractions, and cannot differentiate contractions that will subside spontaneously from those that will lead to delivery. The frequency of contractions does not reflect the force of labour.

External transducers do not measure contractions directly. The most sensitive and sophisticated modern strain gauge is merely recording the effects of a contraction through the muffling effect of the abdominal wall with more 'noise' being added from maternal muscle movement outside the uterus, such as breathing and abdominal movement. Mixed in with maternal movements, from whatever source, will be the movements of the fetus. A large fetal movement will distort the wall of the uterus, so much so that a sudden steep rise of the fundus recorded externally is more diagnostic of a sharp fetal movement than a contraction (Mylks *et al*, 1954). It appears to be an extremely crude measuring device. For the information it gives, it is most certainly not worth sacrificing the mother's mobility and almost necessarily disrupts the very thing it is supposed to be measuring.

I have repeated this information from Chapter 4 and laboured the point because it changed obstetric thinking about the nature and purpose of contractions in labour. If Reynolds was correct, maternal position in labour was irrelevant to the course of labour; indeed so heavy were the strain gauges that the women had to be immobile on their backs for recording to be possible at all. Before the fundal pacemaker theory was accepted, obstetric opinion was that: 'In the second stage of labour the general intra-uterine pressure acts as a guiding force, keeping the child in the best position for delivery.' I would go further and think that contractions are also a guiding force in early labour, though in 1932 the stretch-contract mechanism had yet to be discovered. However, once the notion of a guiding force was lost, maternal position became immaterial.

Bruce Mayes' *A Textbook of Obstetrics* was published in 1950. Discussing ways of recognising progress in labour he was still able to write: 'During the first stage as the pains become worse the woman often emits a low moaning sound which for many years was recognized by doctors and midwives as of diagnostic value.' The phrase 'for many years was recognized' is telling; already the subjective assessment of labour by listening to the sounds women make was becoming obsolete. With the dawn of tocography the subjective diagnostic value of the sounds the mother made would go unheard.

Although multi-site tocography was misleading, recording

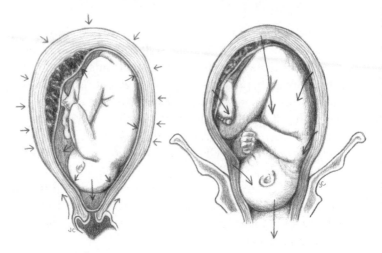

Figure 44: Left: Direction of contractions. Intra-uterine pressure. Early first stage, intact waters, lower segment passive. *Right:* Direction of contractions in the second stage of labour. Direct uterine pressure, full dilatation, membranes ruptured, fetal axis pressure inevitable (after Berkeley and Dupuy, 1932).

from a single site near the fundus was thought to be an objective measurement of contraction strength and frequency. Graphs of intrauterine pressure did correlate quite well with graphs of abdominal stretch in terms of the overall length of the contraction, although peaks could be seen in different places for the same contraction when simultaneous recordings were made. The tocodynamometer was, and still is, a crude strain gauge:

> The only information from the tocogram which can be considered as reliable is a number of the contractions detected. Quantitative parameters describing contractions like duration or strength can be estimated with quite poor accuracy. Thus, tocography is mainly treated as a technique useful for the control of labour progress. This limitation has been confirmed by comparing the external tocography with the intrauterine pressure measurement. (Matonia *et al*, 2006)

I must, however, acknowledge that Matonia had an alternative agenda – to introduce electromyography.

The scientific analysis of the progress of labour required, wherever possible, replacing human observation with numbers. Cardiotocography (CTG) combined tocography with a simultaneous recording of the fetal heart rate. Obstetricians thought they could now see how well the fetus was coping with his mother's contractions; the graph of the fetal heart could be compared with the graph of the abdominal pressure gauge. Big business became involved. CTG machines cost thousands of dollars and there was money to be made from recommending fetal monitoring for all births. Hewlett Packard developed the first commercially available cardiotocography machine in 1968. It was no longer necessary to observe the mother – indeed she would not be believed if she reported having a contraction that was not visible on the print-out (contractions which failed to push the uterus outwards would not register). The machine could take over and the caregivers could look at the machine instead. The woman was in danger of being seen as merely a contracting uterus. The progress of mother and baby could now be monitored with minimal human interaction. Caregivers could become machine minders and technicians.

The fetal heart slows down just after a contraction when blood supply to the placenta is reduced. What matters is how quickly the fetal heart recovers from the effects of a contraction. If caregivers relied on external monitoring they could be mistaken. A benign 'early deceleration' taking place after a peak recorded by an internal pressure balloon could be mistaken for a 'non-reassuring' 'late deceleration' from the graphic output of an external transducer which failed to pick up the later peak. This mismatch could account for babies delivered by caesarean section in perfect health despite monitors showing fetal distress.

The term electronic fetal monitoring (EFM) has now replaced the term CTG. Strain gauge transducers are no longer so bulky but EFM remains a significant barrier to freedom of movement in labour. Although monitoring at a distance by radiotelemetry has been available since at least 1976 (Flynn, 1976), women are usually still tethered to a machine and denied mobility. When fetal alignment is suboptimal, restricting the mother's position will take away any chance there might be of

Midwives talking about tocography

The following quotes were taken from allnurses.com/ob-gyn-nursing/can-someone-explain-390952.html:

'I've had patients having moderate to strong contractions (that I palpated) that showed absolutely zip on the monitor. The real hard part (at least for me) is getting docs to believe me when I say she's contracting and nothing's showing up on the EFM.'

'Unless you have INTERNAL uterine pressure monitoring ... the intensity of the contraction is pretty meaningless. The external toco is affected by how tight it is applied. Apply it tightly and the height of the contraction "appears" higher (stronger) ... apply it loosely, and the height will be lower ("appear" milder). The external toco is good for duration, and frequency of contractions ... but not all that useful for accurate measurement of intensity.'

'As far as tocodynamics are concerned there can really be no "normal". I tell every labor patient and most of my triage patients that the height of the "hills" means absolutely nothing to me when I look at a strip. There are so many extraneous variables it is not even funny. For example. Position of the toco, position of the baby, position of the mother, size of the baby, size of the mother, thickness of the uterine wall, thickness of the fat layer, how tightly the straps are applied, how old the toco is, how sensitive the toco is, how old the monitor is and how sensitive the monitor is.'

'The only thing I care about with external monitoring is when are the contractions happening and what the fetal heart rate does when one happens. I can get that information with my hand better than a toco.'

correcting it through changing position. The belt itself may be placed so tight that it prevents some fetal movement or prevents a contraction spreading. The result may well be the pain of uncoordinated contractions which is then removed via epidural anaesthesia, taking away all cues to the mother to move to alleviate pain. EFM is necessary when a mother has an epidural since she can no longer feel her contractions.

The NICE Guideline *Intrapartum Care* (CG55) is aware that EFM restricts women's mobility but seems unaware of the consequences. NICE states that EFM is advised for abnormal fetal heart rate – despite the fact that the change in maternal position is likely to make the matter worse because of aortocaval compression, pressure on the maternal blood vessels (Kinsella *et al*, 1992).

Continuous fetal monitoring has been researched *ad nauseam*; trial after trial of low-risk women has shown that it increases the caesarean section rate without having any effect on perinatal mortality. This is not really surprising. Unless a woman has an epidural in place, external monitors provide far less information than a midwife can gain from watching and listening to women and listening in to the fetal heart. Monitors plot only the effect of contractions on the abdominal wall and an approximation of the fetal heart rate calculated from ultrasound signals. Midwives at a mother's side get a far clearer picture of how a woman is coping with her labour, and listening to the fetal heart sounds directly through a Pinard stethoscope allows a better picture of how the baby is coping with labour. The knock-on effect of such a liberal use of EFM is the loss of these midwifery skills and yet intermittent auscultation is still as good as EFM.

The latest Cochrane review of randomised controlled trials of fetal monitoring concludes:

> Overall, there was no difference in numbers of babies who died during or shortly after labour (about one in 300) (low quality evidence). Fits in babies were rare (about one in 500 births) (moderate quality evidence), but occurred less often when continuous CTG was used to monitor the baby's heart rate. There was no difference in the rate of cerebral palsy (low quality

evidence); however, other possible long-term effects have not been fully assessed and need further study. Continuous monitoring was associated with significantly more deliveries by caesarean section (low quality evidence) and instrumental vaginal births (low quality evidence). Although both procedures carry risks for mothers, these were not assessed in the included studies.

There was no difference in numbers of cord blood acidosis (very low quality evidence), or women using any drugs for pain relief (low quality evidence) between groups.

Compared with intermittent CTG, continuous CTG made no difference to how many women had caesarean sections or instrumental births. There was less cord blood acidosis in women who had intermittent CTG but this result could have been due to chance. (Alfirevic *et al*, 2017)

This evidence should have been enough to place reasonable limits on continuous monitoring, yet it has made little or no difference to labour ward protocols; women are still warned that their baby will die if they refuse continuous monitoring (Murphy Lawless, 1998; Dagustun, 2012).

Apart from a possible role in maternal reassurance, EFM is never performed for the benefit of the mother. The psychological effect is to distance her from the support of her partner and her midwife. There is a tendency to watch the machine instead of supporting the mother. The discomfort caused by preventing her from adopting comfortable positions for labour and birth is discounted, as is the increased risk of surgical delivery which inflicts the iatrogenic harm (harm caused by medical intervention) of an incision into her uterus. Neither is it carried out for the benefit of her baby, who is more likely to suffer iatrogenic harm from forced surgical delivery. The potential harms include respiratory distress syndrome and scalpel injuries for those born by caesarean section, and injuries caused by forceps or vacuum deliveries. EFM might be convenient for obstetricians who might feel that they can get a more objective picture of what has gone on in their absence from the print-out of a machine, whereas midwives record the progress of labour in the clinical notes and on partograms. It is this 'objective' print-out, however, that is the chief reason for the continued use of

EFM. Clinicians, and later their managers and lawyers, jumped at the chance to have a machine-written record of labour and in the USA EFM is even used in normal labour. The paper record of the progress of a labour can be used in court by lawyers on both sides of the case in an attempt to prove or defend alleged malpractice. As Goer (2013) points out there are plenty of expert witnesses ready and willing to argue whichever side of the case suits their pocket. Ironically, the means of measurement itself was to become a reason why women were confined to the bed, which slows labour and leads to intervention and the associated iatrogenic, harm which leads to law suits.

Pharmaceutical technology

Oxytocin

But the spectre of litigation was still in the future when CTG/ EFM was introduced. CTG had emerged out of studies of the hormones involved in labour and was then used to measure the effects of hormonal intervention in labour. Oxytocin was first synthesised in 1953. In 1960 physiologists doubted the wisdom of supplying the uterus with synthetic oxytocin, calling this intervention 'pharmacological accouchement forcé' (Csapo, 1961), but by the end of the decade, obstetricians were starting to embrace it wholeheartedly. Initial advice was for an obstetrician to be present during oxytocin-induced labours, but as more and more women were induced this soon became impractical and instead CTG became a requirement. Oxytocin was also used to augment (speed up) slow labour. Not all obstetricians were happy with this; it became known as 'daylight obstetrics'.

In 1974 the NHS had recently taken over responsibility for all births, and hospital birth had become the norm. Hospitals must have been struggling to cope with the increased demand for space in the labour ward.* In the 1970s induction and

---

* This is still a problem today; it is solved by restricting access to the labour ward, by sending women home again if they are not far enough advanced in labour – so that too many end up giving birth in hospital car parks – and by closing the ward and telling women to go to a different hospital.

acceleration of labour were used to try and make the most efficient use of available facilities; induction of labour may have been an attempt to even out births over the course of the day and the working week and labour was accelerated so that women spent fewer hours in labour wards. However, this led to outcomes that worried some clinicians. In the autumn of 1974 Liston and Campbell reported concerns about using oxytocin in labour. They reviewed 628 consecutive deliveries in Aberdeen and noted that oxytocin use seemed to be associated with fetal distress, with babies having lower five-minute Apgar scores (a measure of the baby's well being one minute and five minutes after birth) and a greater likelihood of admission to the special care nursery. (This early study is also interesting in that the co-author was a mathematics lecturer and the associations were found by computer using punch hole technology.) Kelly *et al* (1974) responded to that study in a letter to the *BMJ*, pointing out that the amount of oxytocin infused was way beyond physiological levels. They went on to say:

> In some circles the ultimate aim seems to be to cut the induction-delivery interval to 12 hours and virtually to close the labour ward at night. It is not clear in whose interest this time schedule is devised, whether that of the obstetrician, the midwife, the labour ward or the hospital. Perhaps the great majority of women would welcome such a routine, but there is a minority of thinking women who dislike being treated as 'battery hens' and those number may increase when it becomes known that this oxytocin assault is waged on 100% of women when only 20% fail to go into labour as the result of amniotomy alone ...
>
> There is already a ground swell of rumours concerning damage to uterus and cervix and it has yet to be shown that the clinical results so obtained are better than, or as good as, those achieved in the Dutch domiciliary service, which relies on selection of cases and on midwives rather than gadgets.

'Non-thinking' women would object as strongly to being treated like 'battery hens' if only their voices were heard. I have no doubt that, had Kelly, Theobald and colleagues known that 'ambulation' could have obviated the need for the 'oxytocin assault', they would have encouraged all women to escape from their battery cages and range freely instead of being cooped up in labour! In another letter to the *BMJ*, Geoffrey Chamberlain had suggested that ambulation was a better alternative to oxytocin (Chamberlain, 1974).

Prostaglandins

Prostaglandins were next on the hormonal agenda. They were first synthesised in 1969. In 1971 Karim and Trussell reported attempting to induce labour in 500 women by intravenous infusion of prostaglandins and were successful in all but two cases. Researchers found that prostaglandins were most useful not in labour itself, but only for the induction of labour, ripening the cervix to encourage labour to start. It was found that the best route to administer the hormone was vaginally and that it was a more gentle method of inducing labour than large doses of oxytocin. Prostaglandins are now being given as an outpatient procedure which will have the benefit of enabling women to cope with early labour at home. However, unless the uterus is primed with oestrogen – wired up for labour and sensitised to oxytocin – labour will not start despite repeated doses of prostaglandins.

Induction and acceleration of labour

Soon normal birth in hospital became less and less likely. Now it was necessary to use EFM to identify the fetus suffering from over-zealous intervention, and the caesarean section rate began its inexorable rise. There was no longer any incentive to encourage normal birth. By 1974, 39% of labours were being induced in the UK. With every technical advance doctors had more ammunition to blind everyone with science – the policy makers, the clinicians and the general public. Birth became 'scientific' and had to take place in a laboratory – the hospital. Some mothers objected and a few brave clinicians investigated birth in different positions, finding nothing to object to on safety grounds. The obstetric chair made a brief comeback, acquiring an expensive, futuristic look, but ultimately failed to satisfy clinicians who preferred women to be on their backs or in the lithotomy position. Once artificial oxytocin and prostaglandins could be used to induce and speed up labour, obstetricians had no incentive to look further at the mechanisms of normal birth, particularly when caesarean section became a routine and relatively safe operation. Routine operative delivery meant that there was no incentive to keep birth normal and, in places where operative delivery earned an obstetrician more income, there was a financial incentive to intervene.

No doubt induction of labour is clinically useful in a very small number of cases, but forcing a woman's body into labour before it is ready seems to me to be asking for trouble. If the uterus is seen as a battering ram, as the fundal pacemaker model suggests, forcing a baby into a pelvis at whatever angle he is presenting by the liberal use of oxytocin would seem harmless to the obstetrician – if increased pain is also regarded as harmless, which may be the case if women are given epidural anaesthesia. If the older view of uterine function being a 'guiding force' is more accurate then large quantities of oxytocin are likely to do more harm than good. On the other hand if mothers are kept in place in one position by various lines, leads and straps, oxytocin is the only solution. The consequences – a higher rate of vacuum, forceps and caesarean deliveries – are inevitable and should not be regarded as harmless. Whatever measure of harmfulness is considered, whether it is the physical damage to mother and baby, their enforced separation if the baby needs to be admitted to special care, difficulties establishing breastfeeding, a traumatic birth leading to postnatal depression or even post-traumatic stress disorder, all are likely to do more harm than good. The argument for induction of labour for prolonged pregnancy perplexes me. Normal pregnancy is said to last for between 37 and 42 weeks and yet labour is induced routinely at 39 weeks. But now, after 39 weeks of pregnancy, a baby is thought to be under so much stress in the uterus that it would be better for him to be delivered. He is then put through the extra stress of an induced labour and this is thought to be beneficial. From my reading of the literature surrounding induction of labour for prolonged pregnancy (Jowitt, 2012), it seems that doctors' primary fear is of the baby dying before labour starts, what is known as an antepartum stillbirth. While this is devastating for all concerned, and the parents will always be left wondering whether something could have been done, I cannot see the logic of deliberately inflicting more stress on an already stressed baby, if, indeed, he is stressed.

... but longer labour

Ironically, after it became possible to manage labour by the clock, with arbitrary limits to each stage of labour, over the years labour has become longer. Buhimschi *et al* (2003) write:

> Evidence for a temporal trend toward an increase in the duration of labour, more frequent prolongation of the second stage, no deceleration phase, and labours lasting more than 2 hours without perceivable cervical change before 7 cm dilatation is available.

Somewhat bizarrely, they account for this by blaming the mothers, saying that 'Clearly the maternal body mass index and smoking habits have changed over the last 50 years.' They regain no credibility when they observe that: 'Labour induction protocols, indications for operative deliveries, epidural analgesia, management of breech and twin pregnancies also evolved as the population changed.' I would think that labour induction protocols, epidurals and the rest of it were themselves the cause of prolonged labour. Interfering in the natural process of childbirth disrupts normal function and leads inevitably to the cascade of intervention, a vicious circle.

A 2012 study showed that the average length of labour had increased by two and a half hours since the 1960s (Laughon, 2012). A fellow doctor, Michael Cabbad (2012) commented on the paper and thought that delivery room practices explained the findings:

> When patients arrive in active labor, they are placed on monitoring devices that people didn't have in the '60s. They tend to be placed in a labor bed. They get IV fluid hydration, which

tends to slow labor. Women are in bed with limited mobility, not walking, which tends to slow down the labor process.

Conclusion

As each labour hormone was synthesised, clinical trials were performed. As new technology for measuring the fetal heart and the strength of contractions was developed, medical equipment companies concentrated their efforts on producing and selling devices that could be used in labour wards. Birth became big business. The most common reason for mothers and their partners to choose hospital birth is that hospitals have all the technology there in case something goes wrong, yet technology is often the very reason why birth does go wrong, if only because it restricts the mother's mobility so much. Machines cannot help women to give birth. Only people can provide the practical and emotional support that can see a woman through to give birth under her own efforts. Technology can be useful but it can also be overused. It is best saved for when it can do more good than harm.

10 Making birth better

> The barriers to change appear to be complicated and require providers to want to change, and women to be informed of alternative positions during the first stage of labour and delivery. We believe that highlighting the gap between actual practice and current evidence provides a platform for dialogue with providers to evaluate the threats and opportunities for changing practice. (Lugina, Mlay and Smith, 2004)

Despite the rhetoric around women-centred care and choice in childbirth, it is 40 years since most women have had much of a say in where and how they give birth. In the UK we are lucky in that out-of-hospital midwife-led care has remained an option for some low-risk women since the inception of the NHS but today only 14% of women have midwife-led care. From 1970 onwards maternity care was increasingly centralised in obstetric units and now these units themselves are merging to make super-sized units with up to 10,000 births a year. It is difficult in such places to put the needs of women above the needs of the institution. Their very size makes factory-style organisation inevitable. Eighty-six percent of women give birth in obstetric units either by choice, or because there are not enough midwife-led units, or because the midwife-led unit is closed because the labour ward is under staffed, or because they have been labelled 'high risk'.

Most women who choose hospital birth believe the rhetoric of 'just in case' obstetrics, that it is better to be in an environment where 'they have all the technology' and they will be in easy reach of an operating theatre. In early 2014 a medical ethics paper stated that home birth was as risky as failing to use a child car seat (de Crespigny and Savulescu, 2014) and in a Radio London phone-in programme the interviewer reiterated the view that 'birth is safest in hospital' again and again. Why would women put their baby's life at risk for the sake of a lovely fluffy birth experience at home? But it is not until women have given birth in the hospital environment for the first time that they experience the downside of technological childbirth. The technology available in hospital is associated with medical intervention and does not include the low-tech birth equipment that helps women give birth normally. Many clients of independent midwives choose home birth second time around because they felt out of control during their first NHS birth in hospital, because they experienced what is known as the cascade of intervention, which happens on the 'birth by numbers' system, and ended up feeling traumatised.

Safety

The Birthplace Study (2011) looked at what happened to 62,036 low-risk women and their babies in hospital, in birth centres or at home. Out-of-hospital birth proved safer for all mothers; there were no maternal deaths and significantly fewer mothers planning to give birth outside hospital needed surgery. It was as safe for all babies except babies born to first-time mothers who planned home birth. (First-time mothers wanting midwife-led care might perhaps be advised to choose a birth centre.) The study found that low-risk women planning to give birth in obstetric units were more likely to require epidural anaesthesia, vacuum extraction, forceps or caesarean section; they were more likely to need high-dependency care after the birth and their babies were more likely to be admitted to the special care baby unit. Labours were significantly longer in obstetric units, averaging nine hours, whereas in birth centres women took under eight hours to give birth, and home birth took an average of six and a half hours. Birth in obstetric units would have taken even longer were it not so often speeded up with artificial oxytocin (23%) or cut short by instrumental delivery (15%) or caesarean section (11%).

Women do not choose where to give birth on the basis of the ambience and furnishings of the place; they choose on the basis of their perception of safety in different places. The evidence that midwife-led care is safer and kinder has been accumulating year by year until it is virtually unassailable and yet the mainstream media continue to maintain that hospital is safest even though operative deliveries are so common that they are no longer regarded as adverse outcomes. Adverse maternal outcomes are defined in such ways as the need for major blood transfusion or unforeseen high-dependency care, unplanned caesarean hysterectomy to stem major haemorrhage, or the death of the mother. Even though the risk of death to the mother is up to four times higher after caesarean section than after vaginal birth, maternal death is now so rare that the increase in risk to the mother is deemed to be negligible. If a woman wonders whether her operative delivery was avoidable, she is reassured that she has a healthy baby. However, adjusting to life as a new mother is hard enough without also having to cope with the consequences of traumatic birth which can affect a woman's physical and mental health.

The reality of birth position in hospital

The national maternity survey for England for 2013 (Care Quality Commission, 2013) showed that 27% of first-time mothers labouring in hospital had elective or emergency caesarean sections, 23% had instrumental deliveries and only 50% gave birth spontaneously. Half of these mothers will be labelled high risk next time they require maternity care.

The same survey (CQC, 2013) found that 23% had an assisted vaginal delivery, which requires being delivered with legs in stirrups (the 2019 survey does not distinguish between first and second time mothers for mode of delivery), but as many as 48% of first-time mothers reported giving birth in the lithotomy position, implying that half the spontaneous births were conducted in the lithotomy position and most of the rest occurred on the bed. Nineteen percent of spontaneous births in all women took place with the mother's legs in stirrups.

The NICE *Intrapartum Care Guideline 55* states: 'Women should be discouraged from lying supine or semi-supine in the second stage of labour and should be encouraged to adopt any other position that they find most comfortable.' Eighty-five percent of women giving birth vaginally gave birth in a bed, while 8% gave birth in a water or birthing pool. The other options were 'on the floor' (5%) and 'other' (2%). However, 72% of all women, whether giving birth for the first time or not, agreed that they 'were able to move around most of the time to choose the position that made them most comfortable during labour and birth, an increase from 64% in 2010'. Given that the survey included an unknown proportion of mothers who gave birth at home and in birth centres, where women have far more freedom of movement, it looks as though the vast majority of hospital births take place on the bed. But why were mothers also reporting that they could choose positions that made them comfortable 'most of the time'? Perhaps they simply accepted that it is just not possible to feel comfortable during the birth itself, and they had *expected* to give birth in an uncomfortable position on a bed.

Why are maternal outcomes worse in hospital?

Other than the 'cascade of intervention' that occurs in births managed by obstetric protocols, we do not know the precise causes of the increased risks to the mother of hospital birth. There are various factors involved, both physical and psychological. Belief systems may play a part; women choosing out-of-hospital birth may have more faith in their ability to give birth without medical assistance and midwives choosing to care for such women may have more confidence in the natural birth process; they may be better able to support natural birth. Midwives caring for mothers labouring outside hospital will give 'hands off' care, they will refrain from breaking the waters to speed labour up, they will be more patient; if labour is progressing slowly but surely, they will factor in the stress of the transfer itself before deciding to transfer into hospital. In contrast, hospital belief systems see medical, instrumental and surgical interventions as normal procedures which reduce risk.

Women giving birth out of hospital are also more likely to know their midwife, and trust works both ways – if a mother knows her midwife, then the midwife knows the mother. Meeting a mother before labour gives the midwife the advantage of having a prior relationship with her, which can be a great advantage and is described more fully in the book *The Midwife-Mother Relationship* (Kirkham, 2010).

The chances of a woman receiving care from someone she already knows are slim in huge hospitals staffed by doctors and midwives working on shift systems. This is not seen as a problem by the Department of Health (Poulter, 2014).

The reason for the shorter labours and fewer operative deliveries in births planned elsewhere may be quite simply that women's bodies usually work better outside the stressful hospital environment. Grantly Dick-Read was the first to articulate this with his 'fear tension pain' cycle (Dick-Read, 1942) and the physiological explanation concerns the role of stress hormones in labour (Jowitt, 1993; Buckley, 2011). Stress also affects the doctors and midwives in hospital – stressed staff may also be more fearful and more inclined to intervene.

Thus the hospital environment is not good at providing psychological support for women, but neither is it good at providing physical support. The high-tech hospital environment does not usually provide low-tech physical support for women's bodies in labour.

The hospital environment

The hospital environment affects everyone's behaviour. A woman choosing hospital birth has far less control over how birth will be managed than a woman choosing midwifery care in a birth centre or at home. Childbirth is a particularly difficult area of hospital practice because it involves two 'patients', the mother and her baby, both of whom can be harmed by too much or too little intervention or by the cruelty of nature itself. When such harm occurs and, sadly, sometimes it is inevitable, the impact on the family is devastating and the financial penalty on hospitals through litigation is immense. According to Hansard, (record of the proceedings of Parliament, November 2017) 'the NHS spent almost £500 million settling obstetric claims in 2016-17. For every £1 the NHS spends on delivering a baby, another 60p is spent by another part of the NHS on settling claims related to previous births.'

When things go wrong, there is also an emotional impact on doctors and midwives and this will make a difference to the way they practise when they next encounter a similar situation.

It is always a fine line between intervention and watchful waiting, and each midwife and each doctor draws the line at a different place. Doctors see more labours that have 'gone wrong'; midwives see more that go well. We all act according to our past experience, that is part of the human condition, and this is why the clinical evidence for and against every single intervention is so crucial. Doctors also tend to err on the side of intervention because they have been trained to *do* things, and from the earliest of times, midwives have always had to call the doctor when they needed something to be done. Although midwives cannot work safely without surgical back-up, they tend to err on the side of watchful waiting, letting a labour unfold. The Birthplace Study (2011) showed that there is no need for doctors to be involved in normal birth unless a woman needs to be transferred, but when birth takes place in hospital, doctors control how birth is to be managed. Women and midwives have to negotiate their way around obstetric and management guidelines. Labour has become a process to be managed and controlled in an attempt to reduce the risk of adverse outcomes that might lead to litigation. There is little room for flexibility in the way that staff are required to work. There is even less flexibility for women.

How birth progresses in hospital depends so much on other people's behaviour – the culture of the hospital, its staffing levels, its protocols, guidelines and policies, how much doctors trust the midwives, how much midwives trust the doctors – and how much mutual trust there is between management and clinicians. Theoretically, interventions are offered to women and women are at liberty to decline, but if there is an adverse outcome and the midwife is investigated she may be castigated for not being forceful enough in 'persuading' a woman of the need for an intervention (Montagu, personal communication). This process is common enough to have been given a name, 'protective steering' (Levy, 1999).

Even though the rhetoric states that women should give their informed choice and be at the centre of their care, I would argue that this simply is not possible in the hospital environment because the repercussions when something goes wrong are so enormous for all concerned. Informed consent has become just another box to tick. The verb 'to consent' has changed from an active verb to a passive verb. Women no longer consent to treatment, now they are 'consented' for intervention. It has even become an active verb again – but active on the part of the caregiver not the recipient of treatment. I have seen a letter from an obstetrician containing the words, 'I consented her for caesarean section.' Midwives and obstetricians cannot consent women; women have to give their consent. The language used betrays the passivity expected of the woman. Consent should also be 'informed' but if all the benefits of the intervention are listed and none of the risks, then consent is not informed.

In hospital, midwives are aware that their every move is scrutinised both by management and by colleagues. Women can be very judgmental and cruel to each other; midwives who try to make birth as natural as possible can find themselves ridiculed and ostracised by their colleagues. Peer pressure is a very powerful means of forcing behaviour into the cultural norms of a workplace (Jowitt, 2008). Students may learn the theory of 'watchful waiting' in university classrooms, but once they start clinical practice there is strong pressure to be obedient and conform to the hospital culture (Hollins Martin, 2008). It is peer pressure that makes it acceptable practice for midwives to deliver women in the lithotomy position and rare for women to give birth on the floor – despite the recommendations of NICE guidelines.

Large institutions simply cannot feel as friendly and welcoming as small birth centres. Hospitals are brightly lit, there are too many strangers about the place and there is little that can be done to avoid the bustling hospital atmosphere. Labour wards are so busy and security is so tight that some women no longer have the chance to visit the unit before the birth to familiarise themselves with the place. When they are admitted in labour, everything feels new and strange, particularly for a woman who has never been in hospital before. Women are bound to feel apprehensive about an unknown future. The stress hormone system is activated, making labour painful and slow.

The hospital midwife is caught betwixt and between. She works in a stressful environment where labour takes longer on average. She is stuck with a set of obstetric guidelines in a room full of obstetric equipment but containing the bare minimum of midwifery equipment. If care starts out on the bed with routine admission procedures, it is difficult for the midwife actively to promote freedom of movement from the very beginning. If failure to progress is diagnosed, the cascade of intervention starts and the belief that women need doctors for birth becomes self-perpetuating.

What women need

Before the birth women need antenatal education to gain an understanding of how their body works and to enable them to understand the benefits of remaining active and upright in labour. They need to know that they can play an active part in achieving a less painful labour and a normal birth and that this is safest for themselves and their babies. Such information is essential to counteract the near universal images in the media of suffering women lying on hospital beds, wired up to machines and connected to intravenous drips. Women need more than just encouragement to adopt comfortable positions in labour, they need to be informed of the disadvantages of positions which constrict the movements of their uterus and keep their pelvis closed. Antenatal education could introduce them to the low-tech birth equipment that is available in hospitals. An antenatal class involving birth balls would be hilarious and make a good counterbalance to passive listening.

Regina Coppen (2005) performed a randomised controlled trial of the effect of antenatal education, comparing knowledge and outcomes in women who attended a 90-minute session of focused information about birthing positions with those who

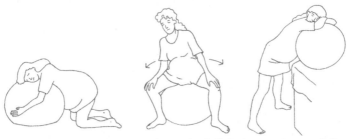

Figure 45: Using a birth ball: *Kneeling with a ball, Sitting swaying on a ball* and *Standing, leaning on a ball.*

attended a general information session on strategies for coping with labour. The women receiving the session on birth position were more informed and had stronger preferences for upright positions, but there was no statistically significant difference in outcomes. Sadly, despite focused antenatal education, Coppen found that midwives had more say in where and how the women gave birth.

During labour all women need the physical and emotional support of a midwife who will remain alongside them in labour and encourage them to labour and give birth in any position they want, whether that be standing, sitting, kneeling, lounging or lying on a bed. Women need a midwife to reassure them that what they are feeling is normal (or to be an advocate by their side if things seem to be going pear-shaped). During labour and birth women need the right type of birth equipment to enable them to prop themselves up and *find for themselves* the

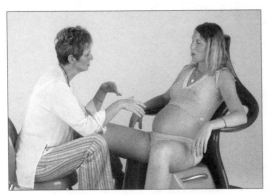

Figure 46: Birthrite birthing seat.

positions which will reduce their pain and let their body work efficiently and effectively. They don't usually get this in hospital unless the pool room is free, and the hospital has enough staff on duty to make a midwife available throughout labour, and there is a midwife on duty who is confident and willing to support a woman labouring in water. Pool rooms are a great advance, but not every woman wants a water birth and women labouring out of water also need an environment designed for giving birth.

Most birth centres have equipment designed for labour and birth; most hospitals lack such equipment and yet women who choose hospital birth, for whatever reason, have just as much of a right to freedom of movement as women choosing out-of-hospital birth. A comfortable environment conducive to normal birth must surely be a basic requirement for all labouring women. The people working in hospital are given the right tools for their jobs but the labouring mother often lacks the right tools for her own work. Most women would be perfectly capable of giving birth without medical assistance if only they had the right furniture and the right midwife. Even

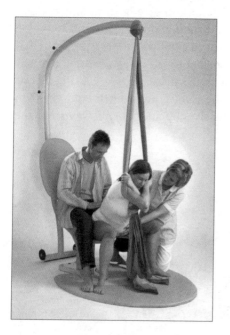

Figure 47: Mother and midwife friendly Febromed equipment designed to facilitate upright birth.

those who choose a hospital birth because they are convinced that they will need an epidural may be pleasantly surprised to find labour more bearable if they can labour off the bed.

What babies need

Babies need to be born gently to a mother who is in the best possible state of physical and mental health. Midwives practising in birth centres and at home know that by caring for the mother you care for her baby. They have always monitored the progress of labour by observation. As well as listening in to the fetal heart after contractions and recording the results (intermittent auscultation), they are aware of the mother's pain, the strength of her contractions, her ability to converse, the noises she makes, her demeanour, the colour of her cheeks, the length of the purple line between her buttocks (Shepherd *et al*, 2010), the coldness of her legs and so on. The progress of labour can even be gauged by maternal position – the nearer to the ground a woman gets, the closer the birth (Horler, 2014). While a labour is progressing the *mother* is caring for her baby.

NICE guidelines say that fetal monitoring is not necessary for low-risk women, and that they do not need even an 'admission trace' at the start of labour, but NICE guidelines are only advisory. It is up to individual hospitals and doctors to decide policy in their own domains. Doctors hope that the CTG print-out will tell them how well the fetus is coping with labour but EFM does not *care* for the fetus, it merely records FHR and contraction patterns. The CTG trace still needs expert interpretation, which is such a complex art that midwives are required to undergo regular refresher courses (Devane, 2005). Information written specifically for women by a doctor on a website designed for patients states,

> There appears to be at best a tenuous connection between cardiotocographic findings, what they signify about the fetal condition and any improvement in outcomes as a result of intervention based upon them. (patient.co.uk)

The worst thing about fetal monitoring is that all too often it puts the woman in bed and turns her into a passive patient. If doctors want to record the progress of labour, hospitals should invest in longer leads or machines which monitor by telemetry. Also the mother can be deprived of emotional support. Both her midwife and her partner may be inclined to look at the machine, not the mother.

I would argue that most babies do not need their mother's labour to be induced. Whole population statistics from the NHS Hospital Episode Statistics (NHS Information Centre for Health and Social Care, 2013) consistently show more assisted deliveries and caesarean sections after induced labour at every stage of gestation. Induced labour always starts with the woman in bed, if only for a vaginal examination and the insertion of a pessary, and mandates obstetric management. Induced labours must be monitored more closely. The cascade of intervention starts even before labour gets going. Again, NICE guidelines say that after induction has started, if all seems well, there is no need for continuous fetal monitoring but hospital protocols may dictate otherwise. It has been suggested that induction of labour is a way of practising 'daylight obstetrics', spreading out births over 24 hours. Most women go into labour at night but hospitals are better staffed during the day. Is it acceptable to fit women's bodies to hospital routines or should we find some other way of making sure every woman has her own midwife when she needs one? Caring for the unborn baby means caring for his mother, avoiding induction which makes her labour harder than necessary, and fulfilling her need for emotional support and physical comfort when her baby and her body are ready for labour.

How can we keep women off the bed?

Throughout this book I have been arguing that the bed itself is the first obstetric intervention in hospital. Once it has been confirmed that women are in active labour, they are introduced to their midwife and taken to a room dominated by a bed. Most women expect to use it, sooner rather than later, simply because it is there. Although there is an expressed desire to promote normal birth and there is plenty of research to show that upright positions shorten labour and reduce the instrumental and operative delivery rates, hospital labour rooms are still designed around the bed. Hospital labour rooms do not look homely enough to encourage women to use the floor. Imagine yourself sitting on the floor during a consultation with your GP and you will get the picture. The message sent out by hospital labour rooms is that the space belongs to the hospital not to the woman and her midwife. There has to be at least a couple of easy chairs and a carpet in any room before it can be viewed as a place where sitting on the floor is acceptable behaviour. Infection control policies mean that labour rooms cannot have carpets but they could have exercise mats, kneeling pads and lots of pillows.

The Royal College of Obstetricians and Gynaecologists, the Royal College of Midwives, NICE guidelines and Cochrane reviews of evidence-based practice, all recommend that women should be encouraged to labour and give birth in upright positions (see Chapter 3), but the advice cannot be taken up unless there is some means of enabling women to maintain upright positions for long periods of time without tiring. Advice about position in labour may be written into guidelines in some obstetric units, but a tick in a box may be enough for a midwife to record that she has offered advice, not that she has actively helped women to adopt alternative positions. The evidence from surveys indicates that women tend to use traditional positions for birth. It is argued that obstetric beds can be manipulated in all sorts of ways to allow different positions, but the bed is usually too high for women to feel 'grounded'. With their heavily pregnant belly, they cannot change positions easily, their body feels unwieldy and they may need hands-on help even to turn over.

Existing furniture

Care in hospitals had always been based around the hospital bed, but in the 1980s, an obstetric bed for every room became the aspiration for all up-to-date maternity hospitals. This may have been a health and safety initiative to save the strain on midwives' backs by enabling them to deliver babies directly in front of the woman instead of being twisted to one side. Obstetric beds in every room may have taken the pressure off operating theatres, which often had a queue of women waiting for a caesarean section; or perhaps they were for the benefit of obstetric anaesthetists setting up an epidural. Whatever the reason, the obstetric bed could be easily converted for forceps or ventouse deliveries by removing the end section and putting the woman's legs in stirrups. It could be wheeled directly into an operating theatre, just yards from the delivery room. But the bed was designed for the dramatic part of labour, the birth itself, not for the needs of women during labour. Women labouring in hospital have the same need for physical support as women labouring elsewhere. Many low-risk women choose hospital birth and both high-risk and low-risk women need purpose-designed furniture.

The central position of the bed in the room is a problem but it is not the only problem. Some birth centres have obstetric beds but still manage to support women in labour without using them; the bed is placed in a corner of the room, and the

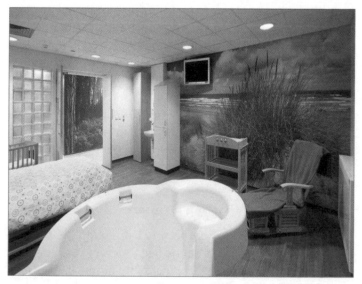

Figure 48: The environment of a birth centre is much more conducive to freedom of movement in labour: Serenity Birth Centre, West Midlands.

birthing pool may take centre stage instead. Birth centres have the advantage of having no fetal monitors and many of their rooms also have a birth pool. There may be a rocking chair and even a sofa as well as equipment specially designed for labour – wall bars, ropes, slings and birth chairs. An expectation of active labour is part of the package. It may not be the bed that is the problem. It may be the mindset of all concerned – the woman, her partner and her midwife.

Whether or not a woman is able to have continuous support from a midwife, the room itself could be designed to cater for women's needs for physical and emotional support and thus promote normal birth. If not, the allocated room may serve to reinforce the more alarming aspects of medicalised childbirth. Unless women have reached the 'point of no return' and they arrive in hospital practically ready to push (i.e. their body has asserted its need to give birth *now*), they need time to acclimatise to the clinical environment before they can follow their instincts to labour and give birth. Women need to feel safe before getting on with their labour. It is common to find that women's contractions slow down or even stop on admission to hospital. This is a perfectly normal hormonal response to an environment that is seen as threatening. The physical environment of the birth room can do much to dispel fear or it can compound it.

If women are fortunate, a labour ward birth room will look like a hotel room, perhaps with a picture or two on the wall. With any luck, the bed will have been pushed to one

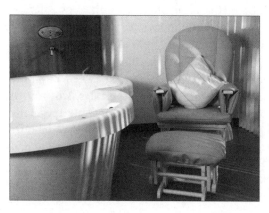

Figure 49: The birthing room in the Halcyon Birth Centre, West Midlands (now, alas, closed).

side and will be at its lowest height; much of the technological equipment will be hidden away out of sight and there will be a birth ball, a bean bag and a floor mat. All this will encourage women to keep off the bed. The room needs to be designed so that women feel comfortable getting down on the floor to labour and their midwives should be happy to support them in whatever position they adopt at whatever stage of labour.

If women are unlucky, the room will contain the technological accoutrements of modern obstetrics: a fetal monitoring machine; a wall full of pipes, wires, switches and buzzers; a couple of drip stands at the ready; and a resuscitaire in the corner. The bed will have been raised up to its highest level for ease of cleaning after the last occupant of the room. All this equipment presents a daunting prospect to the soon-to-be parents. Having been led to expect that it is safer in hospital where they have all the technology, the technology is too difficult to ignore and there is an expectation that it will be used. The bed acts as a magnet. If women are lucky, they will have had initial observations, the first vaginal examination and the rest of it elsewhere, but if not they will have to 'pop up onto the bed' straight away and may never get off it again. Or the bed may be used for an 'admission trace' from the fetal monitor to 'establish baselines'. Although women and their partners may be expecting this and may even feel reassured by an admission trace, NICE guidelines say there is no need for this. It is far better that the monitor should be hidden away out of sight.

Attempts have been made to improve the environment in obstetric units but a birth ball is often the only concession to a woman's need for physical support in an upright position during labour. This is a wonderful piece of low-tech kit which brightens up the birth room (Shallow, 2003), but having a birth ball in every room doesn't seem to be having any effect on the instrumental delivery and caesarean section rates. Do women know how to use it and do midwives demonstrate the many ways that it can be used to support women's bodies in labour? Is there a poster on the wall giving examples? Is a kneeling mat readily available? Are there plenty of pillows?

Improving the birth environment

The easiest thing to be done to improve women's experience in hospital is to make the environment feel less clinically threatening. People already working within the hospital environment will not see it as threatening. An experienced midwife who has worked her whole life in hospital will have become used to the environment. As Marsden Wagner, one time Director of Women's and Children's Health at the World Health Organisation, said at the Australian Homebirth Conference in 2000, 'Fish can't see water'. Hospitals actively need to find out mothers' experience of the hospital environment itself. Comments on patient experience questionnaires would provide a rich source of information, particularly if there was a question directly relating to the labour room environment, its ambience and the equipment available.

Student midwives on their first hospital placement are in a similar position to mothers: they are entering an unknown environment, apprehensive about what the future will hold for them; they would be an excellent source of first impressions. Various architectural partnerships have acquired expertise during the design process of one of the new-build birth centres. Architectural design consultants can be commissioned to assess the current environment, identify problems and suggest ways of improving the feel of the place. They could be accompanied by a new mother who has recently given birth in the hospital to tell of her own experience. Other sources of expertise can come from arts and health charities. The National Childbirth Trust designed a *Creating a Better Birth Environment Audit Toolkit* for exactly this purpose in 2003 to ensure that women have the kind of surroundings and facilities that they need to cope well with labour (NCT, 2003). The NCT also offers a consultancy service.

Having researched the effect of maternal position for this book, I believe that furniture designed especially for labour must be an absolute priority. As well as the fetal monitor, all labour rooms need equipment designed to keep women off the bed. A birth stool reduces intervention; a fetal monitor increases it. Unless there is a highly visible alternative, women will continue to gravitate towards the bed.

I spent hours on the internet just looking at furniture and I came up with a design for a kneeling chair for labour, a piece of furniture that provides physical support favouring the forward-leaning positions that I found so helpful in my own labours; the chair was in effect half a sofa. I spent hours trying out different positions using my stairs, chairs and sofa to get an idea of the ideal heights. On demonstrating a wooden prototype at a Maternity Services Liaison Committee meeting (the MSLC is a patient/staff forum) the men present looked perplexed but the midwives, could see its possibilities immediately and thought up other uses, including a place for the first breastfeed. One suggested that if it was a bit bigger it could double up as somewhere for the partner to sleep but I wanted it to be small enough to fit into any labour room and I wanted it dedicated to women's needs. It had to be immediately apparent that it was for the woman to use, not her partner. Another midwife pointed out that it should be packaged with a low chair for the midwife.

Whatever equipment there is, the midwife allocated to the labouring woman will have most influence on whether or not

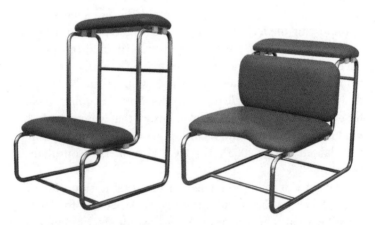

Figure 50: The Osborne kneeling chair designed by the author to provide support at different heights for standing, upright kneeling and all-fours positions – or however a woman wants to use it. www.birthupright.co.uk.

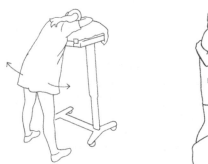 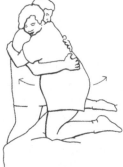

Figure 51: Forward-leaning positions: *Standing, swaying with a tray table* and *Kneeling, rocking with partner support.*

it gets used. Midwives need to demonstrate ways of using birth equipment to show women the possibilities, but they also need to emphasise that women can use any item of furniture however they like. All sorts of positions can be used in labour; there is not an optimal position for birth. Women need to follow their instincts.

I have tended to use the term 'upright position' as a shorthand but anecdotal evidence shows forward-leaning positions are often helpful in labour. Penny Simkin and Ruth Ancheta's book *The Labor Progress Handbook* shows many imaginative ways of using available furniture (it is significant that Penny trained as a physiotherapist before becoming a childbirth educator. Physiotherapists have a totally different way of looking at the body).

Changing midwives

Midwifery training needs to have as much emphasis on helping women to find comfortable positions as it does in competency in performing a vaginal examination or interpreting a CTG print-out. All midwives need training in listening to the fetal heart with women in different positions and they all need to feel comfortable caring for women labouring in water – and they need to be physically comfortable themselves.

Regina Coppen, a midwife who researched position in labour, found that the more experienced the midwife, the greater the propensity to deliver in the supine position (Coppen, 2005). While newly qualified midwives and students in hospital may be happy to help a woman give birth in whatever position she chooses, older midwives may suffer from back problems, perhaps brought about by too much crawling around on the floor earlier in their careers.

Some midwives retain their passion for woman-led childbirth throughout their careers but many have to leave the hospital environment to practise it. Virginia Howes, an independent midwife, has remained true to her calling to support women in whatever position they choose. She says:

> Nicky's was the first ever birth I attended as a newly qualified midwife. I remember her birth and I have written about it in my book *The Baby's Coming* (Howes, 2014). Nicky remembers the senior midwife coming into the room and seeing her standing by the bed pushing said,
> 'Get your woman on the bed, Virginia'.
> 'This woman is birthing her baby how she wants to – and that is standing,' I replied.

This exchange on a social media site prompted another seasoned midwife, Dot Parry, to relate a story from her own days of gaining confidence as a newly qualified midwife:

> My first 'confidence case' involved my mentor tutting about the sterile field and the trolley and the registrar coming in and declaring, "How can I do a forceps delivery with the woman on the floor?" The woman told them to get lost and gave birth to her baby on a mat on all fours on the floor. There was a comment to the registrar about where she could stick her forceps too …

It is an uphill struggle to change hospital practice. However, some obstetricians are learning that birth needs to take place in the right environment. Amali Lokugamage, a consultant obstetrician, wrote about being transformed by her own pregnancy and the birth of her baby (2013). She has come to believe that, given the right environment, most women would be able to let labour unfold.

The physical and psychological environment can be made conducive to labour unfolding or can stop the process in its tracks. So much depends on the initial encounter between mother and midwife. NICE guidelines say that healthcare professionals and other caregivers 'should establish a "rapport" with the labouring woman, asking her about her wants and expectations for labour, being aware of the importance of tone and demeanour, and of the actual words they use.' As well as ascertaining the woman's wants and expectations, midwives need actively to encourage women to stay off the bed. The idea of the bed is so deeply engrained in the hospital culture and in the public's mind that getting rid of it altogether would not be considered feasible. In 1997, Regina Coppen wanted to do an observational study to look at how midwives cope with the care and delivery of mothers in the presence or absence of a delivery bed but the idea was abandoned because it was thought that some staff and some mothers would not be able to cope with delivering a baby without a bed.

Midwives need to work alongside women once more, getting them to make the best of their own resources, encouraging them to relax and to move about. This midwifery philosophy does not suit the hospital culture and is difficult to sustain over the long term. One quarter of newly qualified midwives think they will survive the hospital system no longer than ten years.

We need more midwives in our hospitals. Some of the stress of entering an overtly clinical environment should be alleviated once a woman is able to settle into her own room with her own midwife but the parents-to-be need a midwife who is not rushed off her feet. The NHS aims to provide one-to-one care throughout labour but the Birthplace Study (2011) found that women in obstetric units had a midwife present for only two thirds of the time. The 2013 Maternity Survey (Care Quality Commission, 2013) found that women who reported being left alone by midwives or doctors at a time when it worried them were more likely to have an instrumental delivery or emergency caesarean section. The number of midwives has not kept up with the higher birth rate and midwives are leaving the maternity services because they can no longer cope with the stress of working in such an environment. Midwives often have to care for more than one woman at a time in hospitals which are bursting at the seams because of hospital closures elsewhere. If the midwives cannot stand the environment, how must the women feel?

The Government's response is always to say that there are more midwives in training but this is disingenuous; it does not address the problem of the current shortage of midwives. Some hospitals are simply unable to recruit enough midwives. On the other hand, obstetric manpower in proportion to the number of childbearing women has increased throughout this century in the UK (OECD, 2013). This is reflected in the statistics of the person 'conducting the delivery' which shows that 40% of babies born in hospital in 2012 were delivered by doctors (up from 24% in 1990) and 60% by midwives (down from 76% in 1990) (HSCIC Maternity statistics 2013). If the NHS can afford more obstetricians, it can afford more midwives.

Changing the culture of hospital birth

Gradually, more birth centres are being built on the same site as obstetric units so that more women can have midwifery care, transferring easily to obstetric care if medical help is needed, but until there are more places where women can have midwife-led care, hospitals need to do more to support women to increase their chance of normal birth.

Writing in the *Sunday Telegraph* in 2014, David Prior, chairman of the Care Quality Commission, called the NHS a monumental paradox:

> It is an organization built upon wonderful values and an almost Panglossian confidence that people – especially doctors and nurses – will behave well, work hard and always act in the best interest of patients. And yet, parts of the NHS have developed a culture that doesn't listen – or worse, that stigmatises and ostracises those who raise concerns or complaints. … it tolerates and institutionalises outdated working practices and

old-fashioned hierarchies … Perhaps most crucially, we need to change the culture … that means looking holistically at the performance of hospitals, using measures that matter to patients and that continuously improve performance.

The Care Quality Commission is asking new mothers the right questions and their answers highlight the dominant bed-based philosophy of hospital birth. I believe women's answers regarding choice of position reflect their expectations. Women expect to labour in a bed and expect to give birth to their babies with their legs in stirrups. People may laugh at the thought of birth on all fours, but looking at it dispassionately, which is the more undignified, giving birth on all fours or giving birth in the lithotomy position? Both are equally inelegant but one position benefits both mother and baby and works with nature while the other acts against the one force none of us can do anything about, the force of gravity.

Towards a new physiology of birth

We need to look further at the physiology of birth at the human level by simple observation and by listening to women and midwives. Physiology research has drilled down so far into what happens at a cellular level that it has lost sight of the whole picture – what happens to the whole woman and her baby. Physiology research takes no notice of how the human mother gives birth in her natural habitat, and only investigates birth in the laboratory conditions of hospital, yet the internet is packed full of women's and midwives' stories of birth, each shedding more light on the physiological miracle that first divides and then reunites mother and baby. This wealth of evidence is completely dismissed by the scientific community yet it probably already contains what could be called the natural history of childbirth if only we would take the trouble to decipher the text. Time and time again women talk of what position they adopted, how they moved, where the pain was, how they coped, what noises they made. They also speak of the joy and empowerment that sets them off on the right foot for motherhood. So much of this is denied to women who labour

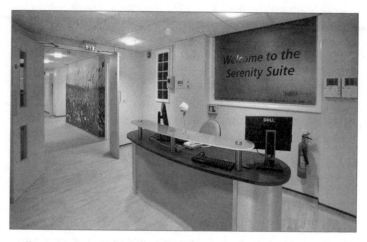

Figure 52: Serenity Birth Centre. A warm welcome.

in hospital. We have enough evidence of what happens in the controlled laboratory of hospital birth. Maybe it is time to analyse systematically women's own accounts to piece together a scientific account of how women's bodies work in labour and learn how to support women in labour so that they can say they have done it themselves.

Hospitals need to rethink the birth environment, invest in screens to hide the technology and invest in furniture and aids to promote freedom of movement, not forgetting the needs of their own staff to have furniture which allows them to alter their own posture to suit the women instead of *vice versa*. Hospital midwives need encouragement to promote freedom of movement for women and to become comfortable with helping women to give birth in different positions. Doctors need to add the 'P' of position to their own mnemonic and realise that improved maternal positions will increase the 'powers', widen the 'passage' and oxygenate the 'passenger'. They may even start to prescribe upright position instead of artificial oxytocin for a mother with a stalled labour. If doctors are so enamoured of fetal monitors, they could replace old fashioned fetal monitors which tether women to the bed with telemetric fetal monitors, transmitting the data to a different room for one of their own number to interpret, letting the midwife get on with her job of being alongside women in labour.

Change is slow and measured in generations rather than years. It took 300 years to get most women into hospital to be delivered on the bed or the operating table. We can but hope that it won't take 300 years to get them off it again.

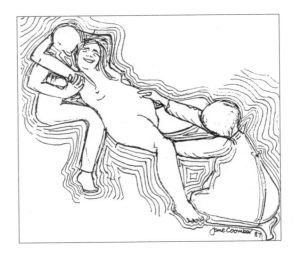

Acknowledgements

This book represents one half of a project that has consumed my life for the past ten years, encouraging women to labour and give birth off the bed. The book outlines the theory behind the Osborne kneeling chair I have designed to help women find comfortable positions for labour. The chair is now available from birthupright. co.uk. Without the help and encouragement of my radical midwife friends, neither project would have seen the light of day. However, I am not a midwife and I take full responsibility for any errors and would welcome enlightenment.

The illustrations were a huge challenge. I must acknowledge the enormous help I had from Jane Cooper and Robert Jowitt for some of the more outlandish figures. They both spent hours trying to extract three-dimensional concepts out of my head and onto paper, fitting imaginary tubes and balloons into various orientations of the pelvis. None of us has trained in anatomy, and the drawings are not to scale, but we hope the images help to illuminate the text. Similarly, Pete Bradley made the most amazing video of a chimp pelvis morphing into the human female pelvis (apologies for the superfluous tail) and a few stills from this appear on on pages 110-111 to illustrate my new biomechanical theory of the reversal of uterine quiescence. Working with composite materials (fibreglass) in designing the chair, and working with Pete to make the animation, both helped to illuminate further the biomechanics of uterine function. Other illustrations come from far and wide. Penny Simkin and Ruth Ancheta kindly allowed me to use drawings from *The Labor Progress Handbook* and other midwives contributed, including Monika Boenigk, Jane Coomber, Kathryn Gutteridge, Sarah Montagu and Jean Sutton. Febromed and Birthrite kindly provided photographs of modern equipment. Some pictures came from complete strangers, intrigued to know why I would need such an image for a book about birth. Thanks to Ceredigion Museum, Karen Gardiner, Stefanie Grübl, M and MD Furniture, Martin-Baker, 'Travis' and Museo Nacional de Antropología, Mexico, and H J Wollersheim.

My long-suffering offspring, Kathleen, John, Robin and David, and my friends, particularly members of the Longdown Ladies, gave me moral support, encouragement and practical help.

Finally, Martin, Sue and Zoë at Pinter & Martin and my editor, Debbie, displayed endless patience. I cannot thank them enough for having confidence in me and faith that this book will spark a debate about the physical needs of women in childbirth.

Image credits

Figure 1 Permission sought. Figures 2, 3, 5 Labor of Primitive Peoples, George Julius Engelmann, 1883. Figure 4 © Midwifery Matters. Figure 6 © Karen Gardiner. Figure 7 © Ceredigion Museum. Figure 8 Practica Maior, Giovanni Savonarola, 1550. Figure 9 The Rosegarden for Pregnant Women and Midwives, Eucharius Rösslin, 1513. Figures 10, 11, 18 © Robert Jowitt. Figure 12 By kind permission of M and M Furniture UK. Figure 13 Unknown. Figure 14 © BirthRite. Figure 15, 27 © Margaret Jowitt. Figure 16 © Shutterstock/Redav. Figure 17 © Martin-Baker Aircraft Co Ltd. Figure 19 © Sarah Montagu. Figures 20, 21, 22 © De Gruyter/Journal of Perinatal Medicine 1975 Mendez Bauer Effects of Standing Position on spontaneous uterine contractility and other aspects of labour. Figure 23, 25, 27, 30, 38, 43 © Margaret & Robert Jowitt. Figures 24, 34, 36, 39, 40, 42, 44 add © Jane Cooper. Figure 26 © Springer-Verlag, Abdominal EHG on a 4 by 4 grid: mapping and presenting the propagation of uterine contractions. Karlsson, B. (et al) 11th Mediterranean Conference on Medical and Biomedical Engineering and Computing 2007. Figure 28, 50 Pete Bradley. Figures 29, 45, 51 Line drawings by Shanna Dela Cruz, copyright Ruth Ancheta 1994, 1999, 2011, reprinted by permission from Simkin, P. & Ancheta R. (2011.) Labor Progress Handbook: Early Interventions to Prevent and Treat Dystocia. Oxford: Wiley-Blackwell. Figure 31 Stefanie Grübl, Vielfältige Materialien. Figures 32, 33 By kind permission of Dr Hans-Juergen Wollersheim. Figures 35, 37, Gray's Anatomy, 1918. Figure 41 © The Practising Midwife issue 3, no. 4, 32-34, 2000, Birth Without Active Pushing Jean Sutton. Figure 46 © BirthRite. Figure 47 © Febromed Figure 48, 52 By kind permission of Serenity Birth Centre, West Midlands, SWBH NHS Trust. Figure 49 By kind permission of Halcyon Birth Centre, West Midlands, SWBH NHS Trust. Figure 50 ® design Margaret Jowitt. Illustration on page 203 © Jane Coomber.

References

Adachi K, Shimada M, Usui A (2003). The relationship between the parturient's positions and perceptions of labor pain intensity. *Nursing Research* 52 (1): 47-51.

Albers L (2007). The evidence for physiologic management of the active phase of the first stage of labor. *Journal of Midwifery and Women's Health* 52: 207-215.

Alfirevic Z, Devane D, Gyte GML (2013). Continuous cardiotocography (CTG) as a form of electronic fetal monitoring (EFM) for fetal assessment during labour. *Cochrane Database of Systematic Reviews* 2013, Issue 11. Art. No.: CD006066.

Anderson H, Barclay ML (1995). A computer model of uterine contractions based on discrete contractile elements. *Obstetrics and Gynecology* 86 (1): 108-111.

Anderson T (2002). Out of the laboratory: back to the darkened room. *MIDIRS Midwifery Digest* 12 (1): 65-69.

Andrews CM, Chrzanowski M (1990). Maternal position, labor, and comfort. *Applied Nursing Research* 3 (1): 7-13.

Armstrong P, Feldman S (2007). *A Wise Birth*. Pinter and Martin, London.

Association of Radical Midwives (2013). *A New Vision for Maternity Care*. Association of Radical Midwives, Morpeth, Northumberland.

Bakker PC, Kurver PH, Kuik DJ, Van Geijn HP (2007). Elevated uterine activity increases the risk of fetal acidosis at birth. *American Journal of Obstetrics and Gynecology* 196 (4): 313.e1-6.

Balaskas J (1983). *Active Birth*, Unwin, London.

Banks AC (1999). *Birth Chairs, Midwives and Medicine*. University Press of Mississippi, Jackson Mississippi.

Baskett TF (2009). The History of Vacuum Extraction. Available from: vaccaresearch.com/Free_Clinicians_Resources.htm.

Batra S (1987). Increase by oestrogen of calcium entry and calcium channel density in uterine smooth muscle. *British Journal of Pharmacology* 92: 389-392.

Bauer M, Mazza E, Nava A *et al* (2007). In vivo characterisation of the mechanics of human uterine cervices. *Annals of the New York Academy of Sciences* 1101: 186-202.

Berkeley C, Dupuy G (1932). *Pictorial Midwifery*. Ballière Tindall, Edinburgh.

Birthplace Study Collaboration Team (2011). Birthplace in England Research Programme (Birthplace Study). All reports accessible at www.npeu.ox.ac.uk/birthplace.

Bishop EH (1964). Pelvic scoring for elective induction. *Obstetrics and Gynecology* 24: 266-268.

Blackwell SB, Grobman WA, Antoniewicz L *et al.* (2011). Interobserver and intraobserver reliability of the NICHD 3-tier fetal heart rate interpretation system. *American Journal of Obstetrics and Gynecology* 205 (4): 378.e1-5.

Bloom SL, McIntire DM, Kelly A *et al* (1998). Lack of effect of walking on labor and delivery. *New England Journal of Medicine* 339 (2): 76-79.

Borell and Fernström (1959). Internal anterior rotation of the fetal head: a contribution to its explanation. *Acta Obstetrica et Gynecologica Scandinavica* 38 (1): 103-108.

Buckley S (2002). Ecstatic Birth: The hormonal blueprint of labor. *Mothering* 111, March/April 2002. Available from: www.mothering.com/community/a/ecstatic-birth.

Buckley S (2011). Undisturbed birth. *AIMS Journal* **23** (4): 4-7.

Buhimschi C, Buhimschi I, Malinow AM *et al* (2003). The forces of labour. *Fetal and Maternal Medicine Review* **14** (4): 273-307.

Cabbad M (2012). Women have longer labors now. Available from: www.webmd.com/baby/news/20120330/women-have-longer-labors-now.

Caldeyro R, Alvarez H, Reynolds SRM (1950). A better understanding of uterine contractility through simultaneous recording with an internal and a seven channel external method. *Surgery in Gynecology and Obstetrics* **91**: 641.

Caldwell WE, Moloy HC (1938). Anatomical variations in the female pelvis: their classification and obstetrical significance. *Proceedings of the Royal Society of Medicine*, *32*, Section of Obstetrics and Gynaecology, sectional page 1-30.

Care Quality Commission (2013). The national maternity survey for England for 2013. Available from: www.cqc.org.uk/public/publications/surveys/maternity-services-survey-2013.

Carlson JM, Diehl JA, Sachtleben-Murray M *et al* (1986). Maternal position during parturition in normal labor. *Obstetrics and Gynecology* **68** (4): 443-447.

Chalmers I, Enkin MW, Keirse MJNC (eds) (1990). *Effective Care in Pregnancy and Childbirth* (volumes 1 and 2). Oxford University Press.

Chalmers I, Hetherington J, Newdick M *et al* (1986). The Oxford database of perinatal trials: developing a register of published reports of controlled trials. *Controlled Clinical Trials* 7, **4**: 306-324.

Chamberlain G (1974). Letter: Dangers of oxytocin-induced labour to foetuses. *British Medical Journal* 3: 684.

Chamberlain G, Stewart M (1987). Walking through labour. *British Medical Journal* **295**: 802.

Chan DPC (1963). Positions during labour. *British Medical Journal* 1 (5323): 100-102.

Charles C (1999). How it feels to be a midwife ventouse practitioner. *British Journal of Midwifery* 7 (6): 380-382.

Chen S-Z, Aisaka K, Mori H, Kigawa T (1987). Effects of sitting position on uterine activity during labor. *Obstetrics and Gynecology* **69** (1): 67-73.

Chiossi, G, Costantine, M, Bytautiene, E, Kechichian, T, Hankins, G, Sbrana, E and Longo, M. (2012). The effects of prostaglandin E1 and prostaglandin E2 on in vitro myometrial contractility and uterine structure. *American Journal of Perinatology*, 29(8),

Cibils LA (1972). Enhancement and induction of labor. In: S Aladjem (ed). *Risks in the Practice of Modern Obstetrics*. Mosby, St Louis, Missouri.

Clarke AP (1891). The influence of position of the patient in labor in causing uterine inertia and pelvic disturbances. *Journal of the American Medical Association* 16: 433.

Cochrane A (1979). Quoted in M Enkin: Beyond evidence: The complexity of maternity care. *Birth* **33** (4): 265-269.

COMET Study Group UK (2001). Effect of low-dose mobile versus traditional epidural techniques on mode of delivery: a randomised controlled trial. Comparative Obstetric Mobile Epidural Trial. *Lancet* **358**: 19-23.

Coppen R (2005). *Birthing Positions: Do Midwives Know Best?* Quay Books, MA Healthcare, London.

Cotton J (2010). Considering the evidence for upright positions in labour. *MIDIRS Midwifery Digest* **20** (4): 459-463.

Crawford M, Marsh D (1989). *The Driving Force: Food, Evolution and the Future.*

Heinemann, London.

Cronk M (2014). Personal communication.

Crowley P, Elbourne D, Ashurst H *et al* (1991). Delivery in an obstetric birth chair: a randomized controlled trial. *British Journal of Obstetrics and Gynaecology* **98**: 667-674.

Csapo AI (1961). Defence mechanism of pregnancy. In: G E W Wolstenholme and M P Cameron (eds). *Progesterone and the Defence Mechanism of Pregnancy*. CIBA Foundation, Little Brown and Co, Boston.

Csapo AI (1973). The uterus: model experiments and clinical trials. In: *The Structure and Function of Muscle,* Vol. 2, edited by GH Bourne, 1-90, Academic Press, New York.

Dagustun J (2012). Beware the dead baby card. *AIMS Journal* **24** (3): 11.

De Crespigny L, Savulescu J (2014). Homebirth and the future child. *Journal of Medical Ethics* doi:10.1136/medethics-2012-101258.

Department of Health (1993) *Changing Childbirth. Part 1. Report of the Expert maternity group*. HMSO, London.

Devane D, Lalor J (2005). Midwives' visual interpretation of intrapartum cardiotocographs: intra- and inter-observer agreement. *Journal of Advanced Nursing* **52** (2): 133-141.

Devedeux D, Marque C, Mansour S *et al*. (1993). Uterine electromyography: a critical review. *American Journal of Obstetrics and Gynecology* **169**: 1636-1653.

Díaz AG, Schwarcz R, Fescina R *et al*. (1980). Vertical position during the first stage of the course of labor, and neonatal outcome. *European Journal of Obstetrics, Gynecology and Reproductive Biology* **11**: 1-7.

Dick-Read G (1942, 2nd edn 2013). *Childbirth Without Fear*. Pinter and Martin, London.

Ding W, Yang L and Xiao W (2013). Daytime birth and parturition assistant behaviour in wild black and white snub nosed monkeys. *Behavioural Processes* **94** (5): 8-11.

Donnison J (1977). *Midwives and Medical Men*. Heinemann, London.

Drife J (2002). The start of life: a history of obstetrics. *Postgraduate Medicine Journal* **78**: 311-315.

Dundes L (1987). The evolution of maternal birthing position. *American Journal of Pediatrics* **77** (5): 636-641.

Engelmann GJ (1883). *Labor Among Primitive Peoples*. J H Chambers, St Louis, USA.

Enkin M, Keirse M, Neilson J *et al* (1989). *Guide to Effective Care in Pregnancy and Childbirth*. Oxford University Press, Oxford.

Enkin M, Keirse M, Neilson J *et al* (2000). *Guide to Effective Care in Pregnancy and Childbirth*. Oxford University Press, Oxford.

Evans J (2006). Cervical weeping. *Midwifery Matters* **111:** 25.

Evans J (2012). Understanding physiological breech birth. *Essentially MIDIRS* **3** (2): 17-21.

Flynn A, Kelly J (1976). Continuous fetal monitoring in the ambulant patient in labour. *British Medical Journal* **2**: 842-843.

Flynn A, Kelly J, Hollins G, Lynch PF (1978). Ambulation in labour. *British Medical Journal* **2**: 591-593.

Friedman EA (1954). Primigravid labour: a graphicostatistical analysis. *Obstetrics and Gynecology* **6** (6): 567-589.

Frye A (2004). *Holistic Midwifery: Volume II*. Labrys Press, Portland, Oregon.

Gardosi J, Hutson N, B-Lynch C (1989). Randomised controlled trial of squatting in the second stage of labour. *The Lancet* **8654**: 74-77.

Gaskin IM (2008). *Ina May's Guide to Childbirth*. Vermilion, USA.

Goer H (1999). Does walking enhance labor progress? *Birth* **26**: 127-129.

Goer H, Romano A (2013). *Optimal Care in Childbirth: The Case for a Physiologic Approach*. Pinter and Martin, London.

Gold E (1950). Pelvic drive in obstetrics: an x-ray study of 100 cases. *American Journal of Obstetrics and Gynecology* **59**: 890-896.

Gould D (1998). Assisted birth not assisted delivery. *Midwifery Matters* **78**: 3.

Green J, Coupland V, Kitzinger J (1990). Expectations, experiences, and psychological outcomes of childbirth: a prospective study of 825 Women. *Birth* **17**: 15-24.

Green J, Baston H (2003). Feeling in control during labour: concepts, correlates, and consequences. *Birth* **30**: 235-247.

Green, MH (2009). The sources of Eucharius Rösslin's Rosegarden for Pregnant Women and Midwives (1513). *Medical History* **53** (2): 167-192.

Greer G (1970). *The Female Eunuch*. MacGibbon & Kee Ltd, Great Britain.

Gupta JK, Hofmeyr GJ, Shehmar M (2012). Position in the second stage of labour for women without epidural anaesthesia. *Cochrane Database of Systematic Reviews* 2012, Issue 5. Art. No.: CD002006.

Hall J (2013). Spiritual care: Enhancing meaning in pregnancy and birth. *The Practising Midwife* **16** (11): 26-27.

Haughton S (1886). *Principles of Animal Mechanics*. Longmans Green and Co, London.

Helen E. O'Connell, Kalavampara V. Sanjeevan and John M. Hutson (2005). 'Anatomy of the Clitoris', *Journal of Urology* Vol. 174, 1189–1195.

Hemminki E, Lenck M, Saarikoski S, Henriksson L (1985). Ambulation versus oxytocin in protracted labour: a pilot study. *European Journal of Obstetrics, Gynecology, and Reproductive Biology* **20** (4): 199-208.

Hillier K, Coad N (1982). Synthesis of prostaglandins by the human uterine cervix in vitro during passive mechanical stretch. *Journal of Pharmacy and Pharmacology* **34**: 262-263.

Hingson RA, Edwards WB (1942). Continuous caudal anesthesia during labor and delivery. *Anesthesia and Analgesia* **21**: 301-311.

Hodnett ED, Stremler R, Weston JA, McKeever P (2009). Re-conceptualizing the hospital labor room: the PLACE (pregnant and laboring in an ambient clinical environment) pilot trial. *Birth* 36 (2): 159-166.

Hollins Martin CJ (2006). Are you as obedient as me? *Midwifery Matters* **110**: 11.

Hollins Martin CJ and Bull P (2008). Obedience and conformity in clinical practice. *British Journal of Midwifery* **16** (8): 504-509.

Honnebier MB, Myers T, Figueroa JP, Nathanielsz PW (1989).Variation in myometrial response to intravenous oxytocin administration at different times of the day in the pregnant rhesus monkey. *Endocrinology* 125 (3): 1498-1503.

Horler A (2014). Sharing the skills: supporting birth without the use of vaginal examinations. *North Surrey Midwife* blog: http://northsurreymidwife.blogspot.co.uk.

Horton E, Jones R, Thompson C, Poyser N (1971). Release of prostaglandins. *Annals of the New York Academy of Sciences* **180**: 351.

Howes V (2014). *The Baby's Coming: A Story of Dedication by an Independent*

Midwife. Headline, London.

HSCIC (2013). *NHS Maternity Statistics – England, 2012-13*, Health and Social Care Information Centre. Available from: www.hscic.gov.uk/catalogue/PUB12744.

Jander C, Lyrenas S (2001). Third and fourth degree perineal tears. Predictor factors in a referral hospital. *Acta Obstetricia et Gynecologica Scandinavica* **80**: 229-234.

Jessop F (1989). Sorry, love, it's OP. *Midwifery Matters*. **42**: 21.

Johnstone FD, Aboelmagd MS, Harouny AK (1987). Maternal posture in second stage and fetal acid base status. *British Journal of Obstetrics and Gynaecology* **94** (8): 753-757.

de Jonge A, Rijnders ME, van Diem MT *et al.* (2009). Are there inequalities in choice of birthing position? Sociodemographic and labour factors associated with the supine position during the second stage of labour. *Midwifery* 25(4): 439-448.

de Jonge A, Teunissen T, Lagro-Janssen A (2004). Supine position compared to other positions during the second stage of labor: a meta-analytic review. *Journal of Psychosomatic Obstetrics and Gynecology* **25**: 35-42.

Jowitt M (1993). *Childbirth Unmasked*. Peter Wooller.

Jowitt M (2008). Bystanding behaviour in midwifery: Machiavellian plot or unintended consequence of hospital birth? *Midwifery Matters* **118:** 11-16.

Jowitt M (2012). Should labour be induced for prolonged pregnancy? *Midwifery Matters* **134**: 9-15.

Jowitt M (2018). Electronic fetal monitoring is more important than freedom of maternal position in labour: AGAINST: A biomechanical model of labour suggests that maternal freedom of movement is critical for a good birth *BJOG: An International Journal of Obstetrics & Gynaecology* Volume 125, Issue 7 May 2018

Karim SMM, Trussell RR (1971).The use of prostaglandins in obstetrics. *East African Medical Journal* 48 (1): 1-12.

Karlsson B, Terrien J, Gudmundsson V *et al* (2007). Abdominal EHG on a 4 by 4 grid: mapping and presenting the propagation of uterine contractions. *11th Mediterranean Conference on Medical and Biomedical Engineering and Computing 2007. IFMBE Proceedings*, **16**, 139-143. See: ehg.ru.is/Papers/BKarlsson_MEDICON.pdf

Kelly J, Flynn AM, Studd J, Theobald GW (1974). Letter: Dangers of oxytocin-induced labour to fetuses. *British Medical Journal* **4** (5936): 101-102.

Kemp E, Kingswood CJ, Kibuka M, Thornton JG (2013). Position in the second stage of labour for women with epidural anaesthesia. *Cochrane Database of Systematic Reviews* 2013, Issue 1. Art. No.: CD008070.

Kinsella SM, Whitwam JG, Spencer JAD (1992). Reducing aortal compression: how much tilt is enough? *British Medical Journal* **305**: 539-560.

Kirkham M (2010). *The Midwife-Mother Relationship*. Palgrave MacMillan, Basingstoke.

Kitzinger S (1993). *Ourselves as Mothers*. Bantam, London.

Kitzinger S (2000). *Rediscovering Birth*. Little, Brown and Company, UK.

La Rosa PS, Nehorai A, Eswaran H *et al* (2008). Detection of uterine MMG contractions using a multiple change point estimator and the K-means cluster algorithm. IEEE *Transactions on Biomedical Engineering* 55 (2): 453-467.

La Rosa *et al* (2009). Uterine magnetomyography contractions analysis. Washington University, St Louis, website: www.ese.wustl.edu/~nehorai/research/ra/MMG3.html (online video of magnetomyography).

Laughon SK, Branch DW, Beaver J, Zhang J (2012). Changes in labor patterns over

50 years. *American Journal of Obstetrics and Gynecology* **206** (5): 419.e1-9.

Lawrence A, Lewis L, Hofmeyr GJ, Styles C (2013). Maternal positions and mobility during first stage labour. *Cochrane Database of Systematic Reviews* 2013, Issue 10. Art. No.: CD003934.

Leap N (2000). Pain in labour. *MIDIRS Midwifery Digest* **10** (1): 49-53.

Leap N, Hunter B (1993). *The Midwife's Tale*. Scarlet Press, London.

Lefebvre DL, Piersanti M, Bai XH, Chen ZQ, Lye SJ (1995). Myometrial transcriptional regulation of the gap junction gene, connexin-43. *Reproduction, Fertility and Development* 7(3): 603-11.

Leng G (2018). *The Heart of the Brain, the hypothalamus and its hormones*, MIT Press, Massachusetts and London.

Levy V (1999). Protective steering: a grounded theory study of the processes by which midwives facilitate informed choices during pregnancy. *Journal of Advanced Nursing.* **29**(1): 104-12.

Liggins GM (1969). Premature delivery of foetal lambs infused with glucocorticoids. *Journal of Endocrinology* **45**: 515-523.

Liston WA, Campbell AJ (1974). Dangers of oxytocin-induced labour to foetuses. *British Medical Journal* **3** (5931): 606-607.

Llewellyn Jones D (1990). *Fundamentals of Obstetrics and Gynaecology, Volume 1 Obstetrics*. Faber and Faber, London.

Lokugamage Amali (2012). *The Heart in the Womb*. Docamali Ltd, London.

Lowdermilk DL. *Anatomy and Physiology of Pregnancy*. Available from: www.coursewareobjects.com/objects/evolve/E2/book_pages/lowdermilk/pdfs/208-230_CH08_Lowdermilk.qxd.pdf.

Lugina H, Mlay R, Smith H (2004). Mobility and maternal position during childbirth in Tanzania: an exploratory study at four government hospitals. *BMC Pregnancy and Childbirth* **4**: 3.

Lupe PJ, Gross TL (1986). Maternal upright posture and mobility in labor – a review. *Obstetrics and Gynecology* **67** (5): 727-734.

Makuch MY (2010). *Maternal positions and mobility during first stage of labour: RHL commentary*. The WHO Reproductive Health Library, World Health Organization, Geneva.

Manabe Y, Okazaki T, Takahashi A (1983). Prostaglandins E and F in amniotic fluid during stretch induced cervical softening and labor at term. *Gynecology and Obstetric Investigation* **15**: 343-360.

Marttila M, Kajanoja P, Ylikorkala O (1983). Maternal half-sitting position in the second stage of labor. *Journal of Perinatal Medicine*, **11**: 286-299.

Matonia A, Horoba K, Jezewski J, Kupka T (2006). Monitoring of contraction activity of uterine muscle by the use of abdominal electrohysterography. *Acta of Bioengineering and Biomechanics* **8** (2): 27-35.

Mauriceau F (1668). *Traité des Maladies des Femmes Grosses et de Celles Qui Sont Accouchées*. Paris.

Mayes BT (1950). *A Textbook of Obstetrics*. Australasian Publishing Company.

McCoy King J (1993). *Back Labor No More!!* Plenary Systems Inc, Dallas, USA.

Méndez-Bauer C, Arroyo J, Garcia Ramos C *et al* (1975). Effects of standing position on spontaneous uterine contractility and other aspects of labor. *Journal of Perinatal Medicine* **3**: 89-100.

Merriman S (1816). *A Synopsis of the Various Kinds of Difficult Parturition, with Practical Remarks on the Management of Labours*. Stonehouse, Philadelphia.

Mesiano S, DeFranco E and Muglia L J, (2015). 'Parturition', in: *Knobil and Neill's Physiology of Reproduction* (volume 2), 4th edn Elsevier.

MIDIRS (2008). *Positions in Labour and Delivery*. Informed choice for professionals leaflet. MIDIRS, Bristol.

Milani-Comparetti A (1981). The neurophysiologic and clinical implications of studies on fetal motor behaviour. *Seminars in Neonatology* 5 (2): 183-189.

Miquelutti, MA, Cecatti JG *et al.* (2009). The vertical position during labor: pain and satisfaction. *Revista Brasileira de Saúde Materno Infantil* 9: 393-398.

Morgan E (1997). *The Aquatic Ape Hypothesis*. Souvenir Press, London.

Morrione TG, Seifter S (1962). 'Alteration of the collagen content of the human uterus during pregnancy and post partum involution' *Journal of Experimental Medicine*, 115, 2, 357-365

Morrow C (2013). Preserving normalcy: an interview with Dr Bootstaylor. *Midwifery Today* 108: 50-52.

Murphy Lawless J (1998). *Reading Birth and Death: A History of Obstetric Thinking*. Cork, Eire.

Mylks GW, Radcliffe PA, Radcliffe RW (1954). The gravid human uterus. *Canadian Medical Association Journal* 70 (3): 235-243.

Nagel J, Schaldach M (1983). The non-invasive measurement of uterine activity. In *Non-invasive Measurements*. Academic Press, London.

Naroll F, Naroll R Howard FH (1961). Position of women in childbirth. *American Journal of Obstetrics and Gynecology* 82: 943-954.

National Childbirth Trust (2003). *Creating a Better Birth Environment Audit Toolkit*. National Childbirth Trust, London. Available from: www.nct.org.uk/get-involved/campaigns/pregnancy-birth-campaigning/campaigning-better-birth-environments.

Newburn M, Singh D (2003). *Creating a Better Birth Environment*. National Childbirth Trust, London.

NHS Information Centre for Health and Social Care (2013). *Maternity Statistics 2012-2013*. Available from: data.gov.uk/dataset/nhs_maternity_statistics_england.

NICE (2007). *Clinical Guideline 55: Intrapartum Care: Care of Healthy Women and their Babies*. National Institute of Health and Care Excellence, London.

Nicolaou KC, Sorensen EJ (1996). *Classics in Total Synthesis*. Wiley VCH, Weinheim, Germany.

Odent M (1999). *Scientification of Love*. Free Association Press, London.

Odent M (2013). *Childbirth and the Future of Homo Sapiens*. Pinter and Martin, London.

O'Driscoll K, Meagher D (1986). *Active Management of Labour*, 2nd edn. Baillière Tindall, London.

O'Driscoll K, Meagher D, Robson M (2003). *Active Management of Labour*, 4th edn. Mosby, London.

OECD (2013). *OECD Health Data 2013 Definitions, Sources and Methods Obstetricians and Gynaecologists*. Available from: www.oecd.org/els/health-systems/Table-of-Content-Metadata-OECD-Health-Statistics-2013.pdf.

Olah KS, Gee H, Brown JS (1993). Cervical contractions: the response of the cervix to oxytocic stimulation in the latent phase of labour. *British Journal of Obstetrics and Gynaecology* 100: 635-640.

Osmers R, Tschesche, H, Rath, W, Szeverenyv, M, Suwer, V, Wolker, I and Kuhn W (1994). Serum collagenase levels during pregnancy and parturition, *European*

Journal of Obstetrics & Gynecology and Reproductive Biology (1994). 53, 55-57

Parer JT, King T, Flanders S *et al* (2006). Fetal acidemia and electronic fetal heart rate patterns: Is there evidence of an association? *Journal of Maternal and Fetal Neonatal Medicine* **19** (5): 289-294.

Parry Dot (2014) Personal communication.

Pilbeam D (1972). *The Ascent of Man: An Introduction to Human Evolution.* Macmillan series in physical anthropology, New York.

Piper PJ (1973). Distribution and metabolism. In: *The Prostaglandins*, F J Cuthbert (ed), Heinemann.

Polden M, Mantle J (1990). *Physiotherapy in Obstetrics and Gynaecology.* Butterworth Heinemann, Oxford.

Poulter D (2014). In letter to AIMS member, qouted in *Midwifery Matters* **140**: 2.

Poyser NL, Horton EW, Thompson CJ, Los M (1971). Identification of prostaglandin $F_{2\alpha}$ released by distension of guinea-pig uterus in vitro. *Nature* **230**: 526-528.

Radcliffe W (1947). *Milestones in Midwifery.* Wright, Bristol.

Ragnar I, Altman D, Tydén T, Olsson SE (2006).Comparison of the maternal experience and duration of labour in two upright delivery positions – a randomised controlled trial. *British Journal of Obstetrics and Gynaecology* **113** (2): 165-170.

Read JA, Miller FC, Paul RH (1981). Randomized trial of ambulation versus oxytocin for labor enhancement: a preliminary report. *American Journal of Obstetrics and Gynecology* **139** (6): 669-672.

Reed R (2010). The effective labour contraction: www.midwifethinking

Reid AJ, Harris NL (1988). Alternative birth positions. *Canadian Family Physician* **32**: 1993-1998.

Reynolds JI (1991). Primitive delivery positions in modern obstetrics. *Canadian Family Physician* **37**: 356-361.

Reynolds SM (1949). *Physiology of the Uterus.* Paul B Hoeber Inc, Harper and Brothers, New York.

Reynolds SM (1951). Uterine contractility and cervical dilatation. *Proceedings of the Royal Society of Medicine* **44**: 695-702.

Rigby E (1857). What is the natural position of women during labor? *Medical Times and Gazette* **15**: 345.

Roberts J, Méndez-Bauer C (1980). A perspective of maternal position during labor. *Journal of Perinatal Medicine* **8**: 255-264.

Roberts JE, Méndez-Bauer C, Wodell DA (1983). The effects of maternal position on uterine contractility and efficiency. *Birth* **10**: 243-249.

The Royal College of Midwives (2010). *The Royal College of Midwives' Audit of Midwifery Practice.* RCM, London.

The Royal College of Midwives (2011). *Campaign for Normal Birth: Getting off the Bed.* RCM, London.

The Royal College of Midwives (2012). *Evidence Based Guidelines for Midwifery-Led Care in Labour.* RCM, London.

Royal College of Obstetricians and Gynaecologists (2009). RCOG statement on maternal position during the first stage of labour. Available from: www.rcog.org. uk/what-we-do/campaigning-and-opinions/statement/rcog-statement-maternal-position-during-first-stage.

Russell JGB (1969). Moulding of the pelvic outlet. *Journal of Obstetrics and Gynaecology of the British Commonwealth* **76**: 817-820.

Russell K (2011). Struggling to get into the pool room? A critical discourse analysis of labor ward midwives' experiences of water birth. *International Journal of Childbirth* **1** (1): 52-60.

Savage W (1989). The effect of the attitudes of the obstetrician on the birthing woman. In: *The Free Woman*. E V van Hall and V Eylard (eds), The Parthenon Publishing Group, Carnforth, Lancs.

Savage W (2007). *Birth and Power: A Savage Enquiry Revisited*. Middlesex University Press.

Sayers D (1938). Are women human? Address given to a woman's society, reprinted by Wm. B. Eerdmans Publishing Co (2005).

Schram R (2013). Understanding the role of guidelines in promoting dignity. Presentation at Dignity in Childbirth conference, Birthrights, London.

Shallow H (2003). My rolling programme. The birth ball: ten years experience of using the physiotherapy ball for labouring women. *MIDIRS Midwifery Digest* **13**: 28-30.

Shepherd A, Cheyne H, Kennedy S *et al* (2010). The purple line as a measure of labour progress: a longitudinal study. 10:54 doi:**10**.1186/1471-2393-10-54

'Short Report' House of Commons social services committee (1984). *Perinatal and Neonatal Mortality Report: Follow up Third report from the Social Services Committee, 1983-84* (Chairwoman R Short) HMSO, London.

Shorten A, Donsante J, Shorten B (2002). Birth position, accoucheur, and perineal outcomes: informing women about choices for vaginal birth. *Birth* **29**: 18-27.

Shribman S (2007). In: Maternity Matters: Choice, access and continuity of care in a safe service. Department of Health, London.

Siever JM, Mousel LH (1943). Continuous caudal anesthesia in three hundred unselected obstetric cases. *Journal of the American Medical Association* **122** (7): 424-426.

Simkin P, Ancheta R (2011). *The Labour Progress Handbook*, 3rd edn. Wiley-Blackwell, Oxford.

Simkin P, Bolding A (2004). Update on nonpharmacologic approaches to relieve labor pain and prevent suffering. *Journal of Midwifery and Women's Health* **49**(6): 489-504.

Smellie W (1752). *A Treatise on the Theory and Practice of Midwifery*, D Wilson, London.

Spiby H, Slade P, Escott D *et al* (2003). Selected coping strategies in labour: an investigation of women's experiences. *Birth* **30**: 189-194.

Stewart P, Spiby H (1989). A randomized study of the sitting position for delivery using a newly designed obstetric chair. *British Journal of Obstetrics and Gynaecology* **96**: 327-333.

Sutton J, Scott P (1996). *Optimal Foetal Positioning* (2nd rev. edn.). Birth Concepts, New Zealand.

Sutton J (2000). Birth without active pushing. *The Practising Midwife* **3** (4): 32-34.

Tew M (1990). *Safer Childbirth?* Chapman and Hall, London.

Transform childbirth connection USA May (2013) Transforming Maternity Care (2013). *Listening to mothers III*. Available from: transform.childbirthconnection. org/wp-content/uploads/2013/06/LTM-III_Pregnancy-and-Birth.pdf.

Tully G (2014). Spinning Babies website: spinningbabies.com.

Ullman R *et al* (2010). Parenteral opioids for maternal pain management in labour, *Cochrane Pregnancy and Childbirth Group*. DOI:

10.1002/14651858.CD007396.pub2

Uvnäs Moberg K (2011). *The Oxytocin Factor*, 2nd edn, Pinter and Martin, London.

Walsh D (2007). *Evidence-Based Care for Normal Labour and Birth*. Routledge, London.

Weston (2014). Campaigning for mother centred care. *Midwifery Matters* **140**: 12-14.

Wickham S (2002). The rhombus of Michaelis: the key to normal birth. *The Practising Midwife* 5 (11): 22-23.

Williams EA (1952). Abnormal uterine action in labour. *Journal of Obstetrics and Gynaecology of the British Empire* **59** (5): 635-641.

Williams RM, Thorn MH, Studd JWW (1980). A study of the benefits and acceptability of ambulation in spontaneous labour. *British Journal of Obstetrics and Gynaecology* **87**: 122-126.

Winkler M, Fischer D-C, Ruck P, Marx T, Kaiserling E, Oberpichler A, Tschesche H, Rath W (1999). Parturition at term: parallel increases in interleukin-8 and proteinase concentrations and neutrophil count in the lower uterine segment, Human Reproduction, Volume 14, Issue 4, April 1999, Pages 1096–1100

Wray S (1993). Uterine contraction and physiological mechanisms of modulation. *American Journal of Physiology* **264**: C1-C18.

Young R (2016). Mechanotransduction mechanisms for coordinating uterine contractions in human labor, *Reproduction* 152, 2 R51-61.

Index